Clinical Approach to Ocular Motility:

Characteristics and Orthoptic Management of Strabismus

SECOND EDITION

Ida Lucy Iacobucci, C.O.

Cover design by Aki Yao
Cover photo courtesy of Marc R. Stephens
Learning Design and Publishing, Medical School Information Services
University of Michigan

Updated March 2016

Produced by Learning Design & Publishing
Medical School Information Services

Published by MPublishing, an imprint of Michigan Publishing
University of Michigan Library

ISBN 978-1-60785-440-1

For my parents and sister;
you are always in my heart.

FOREWORD

Ida Iacobucci, CO - recently referred to by her colleagues as the "Golden Orthoptist" - has been a force in the science and practice of orthoptics here at the University of Michigan and around the world for over 50 years. In this second edition of her textbook on the clinical approach to ocular motility, Miss Ida, as she likes to be called, draws on her extensive experience to update the reader on the current theory, science, and practice involving the diagnosis and treatment of common and rarer oculomotor disorders of the brain and oculomotor system.

Soon after joining the staff and later the faculty in the University of Michigan Medical School, she chaired the National Orthoptic Basic Science Course in Ann Arbor for a number of years where she brought the likes of Marshall Parks, Herman Burien, Frank Costenbader, and others together to teach ocular motility and strabismus practice at the highest level to young orthoptics students. This early leadership in the field has continued to the present through her many contributions to orthoptics and ophthalmology in teaching, clinical practice, and research. She is a sought after teacher of basic and advanced ocular motility skills to hundreds of ophthalmology residents (many choosing pediatric ophthalmology and strabismus careers), fellows, and orthoptics students.

Miss Ida has developed advanced clinical care methodology for the treatment of strabismus and diplopia in our most complex and difficult patients, and her research efforts have resulted in important advances in the treatment of intermittent exotropia with alternate occlusion and over minus therapy, in the use of Bangerter Foils for amblyopia treatment and the combination of exercises, prisms, and foils to treat difficult diplopia. Her work has earned not only the respect of her colleagues but also the most important awards in orthoptics; the Scobee Award for training the best graduating orthoptics student and the Lancaster Award for lifetime achievement and contributions to the field.

These pages and chapters are filled with clinical and diagnostic pearls, which are the key to success in this challenging field - all presented in a readable and understandable format.

I recommend this book to all students who care for patients with strabismus and binocular vision disorders, beginning orthoptics students, and ophthalmology residents, as well as more established practitioners, so that they may better understand diagnosis and treatment to improve patient outcomes and satisfaction.

Monte A. Del Monte, MD
Skillman Professor of Pediatric Ophthalmology
Director of Pediatric Ophthalmology and Adult Strabismus
University of Michigan Kellogg Eye Center

PREFACE

I was diagnosed with myelofibrosis in August of 2009. No treatment was available at that time, but I was accepted into a trial study at the University of Michigan Health System in November of 2010 and this experimental therapy saved my life. My cancer is now in remission with chemotherapy and blood infusions.

During this long period of illness I decided to review and update my book, *Clinical Approach to Ocular Motility*, which was published 34 years earlier. New theories have been presented and accepted in the treatment of strabismus and I wanted to include these new theories. Additionally, based on my 50+ years of experience practicing and teaching in the field, I wanted to provide a more detailed description of the various types of strabismus, focusing on the application of Orthoptic treatment.

The first chapter describes the basic tests needed to evaluate the various categories of strabismus. The remaining 11 chapters give detailed characteristics, management, and orthoptic treatment for each specific category.

This book presents an excellent overview for the practicing ophthalmologist and Orthoptist, and is a valuable addition to the required texts in resident programs and Orthoptic training centers.

Ida Lucy Iacobucci
June 2014

ACKNOWLEDGMENTS

Thank you to Monte A. Del Monte, M.D. and Steven M. Archer, M.D., and to all of the faculty and staff in the Pediatric and Adult Eye Clinic at the Kellogg Eye Center at the University of Michigan, which has been my home for more than five decades.

I would like to especially thank my colleague Bruce A. Furr, C.O., Ph.D. for his helpful suggestions and encouragement throughout the process of writing this manuscript. I wish to deeply acknowledge Karen Norman for the hours she dedicated to typing my lectures and to my Orthoptic student, Kathleen Curtin, who assisted with the manuscript through the final steps.

During the course of writing this book, which is a compilation of my lectures to residents and Orthoptic students, many of my residents and Orthoptic students from 2010 to 2014 helped provide suggestions and refine the content. I was so pleased regarding their interest and wish them many happy years in this incredible and rewarding field of medicine.

I am grateful to Jasna Markovac, Senior Director, Learning Design and Publishing, Medical School Information Services at the University of Michigan, for agreeing to publish my book and for introducing me to her colleague, Karen Kost, Associate Publisher. Without Karen's dedication this book would not exist. Karen worked tirelessly and meticulously on my manuscript as well as on the appearance and organization of the final product.

CONTENTS

Chapter 1

BASIC TESTS TO EVALUATE OCULAR MOTILITY

I. Vision Assessment in Children Under Five Years of Age

1. Visual Acuity Timeline:
   - Newborn = 20/600, child will respond to bright lights by squeezing lids.
   - 1 month = 20/400 child will follow a large object of light.
   - 3-5 months = 20/200 child will reliably follow a target in all gazes.
   - 12 months = 20/40 (estimate) hand-eye coordination developing will grab objects.
   - 2-3 years = 20/30 child can identify/match various pictures.
   - 4+years = 20/20 child can reliably identify letters.

2. Obtaining Reliable VA
   - *Always* measure monocularly with adhesive eye patch.
   - Exception: Nystagmus, low vision - use opaque occluder.
   - *Never* use hand to occlude the eye.
   - Don't give up too soon!

3. Preverbal Children

   a) Light
   - Used for children < 2 months.
   - Shine light into each eye and watch response.
   - Blinking, shielding, squeezing eyes, crying – all normal responses.

   b) OKN Drum/Tape-Evaluate Smooth & Pursuit Nystagmus Movements
   - Rotate drum vertically and watch for lid movement upward/downward.
   - Monocular/binocular – horizontal and vertical movements.
   - Used in children under 6-8 months or developmentally delayed.

   c) Mirror/Doll's Head
   - Hold mirror up to baby so they can see their reflection and move it side to side
   - Normal response = baby will follow image in the mirror
   - Move baby's head from side to side, they will keep focus on your face if they can see you

d) Induced Tropia Test
- 12-20 prism used base up, base down or base in.
- Prism placed over one eye while covering the fellow eye as child fixates on near target.
- Cover removed inducing diplopia.
- Watch eye under prism to maintain fixation of target, repeat process with fellow eye.
- Looking for symmetrical response between both eyes.

An abnormal response would be:
- Eye under prism does not pick up fixation.
- Eye under prism initially picks up fixation but quickly reverts to fellow eye.
- The response determines the notation in the chart i.e. FFM, FF(M), FFnoM.

e) Teller Acuity Cards
- Child offered a choice between patterned stimuli (black and white stripes) vs. homogenous background.
- Based on principle that child will choose a more interesting object to view if the pattern is above VA threshold.
- Cards become progressively more difficult.
- Used best in children under 6 months or developmentally delayed.
- May underestimate VA, especially with strabismic amblyopia.
- Cannot be compared to recognition tests like Snellen.

f) Verbal Children
- Allen pictures
- HOTV
- Tumbling E
- Landolt Rings
- Sheridan Gardner
- Leah Figures
- Snellen Letters

g) Linear vs. Isolated Pictures, E's-HOTV or Letters
- Linear acuity is always more accurate than isolated due to secondary crowding phenomenon.
- Crowding bar letters, pictures, and HOTV are considered equally reliable in linear acuity.
- Using isolated letters/pictures is not reliable in detecting amblyopia.
- If child is hesitant with linear acuity, the examiner can point to each symbol or use crowding bars.

II. Ocular Motility

1. Ductions: movement ability measured independently from that of the other eye
2. Versions: parallel movement of both eyes in any direction.
3. Vergence: movement of both eyes in opposite directions to obtain or maintain single binocular vision.
4. Forced Duction: eye passively rotated in the direction to be tested by force in the office.
   - Restriction: shows positive forced duction.
   - Paralysis: shows negative forced duction.
5. Forced Generation: performed in the office, conjunctiva grasped over the muscle to be tested. Patient is asked to slowly move eye in the direction to be tested. Normal force generated 60-80g.
   - Restriction: normal force generated by muscle.
   - Paralysis: decreased force generated.
6. Agonist: muscle that produces a specific movement when contracted.
7. Antagonist: muscle with opposite action of the agonist.
8. Synergist: muscle that assists the primary muscle helper for making a particular eye movement.

EYE MOVEMENT SYSTEMS

1. Saccadic system – all fast eye movements OKN (optokinetic nystagmus) are also the function of saccades.
2. Smooth pursuit system – eyes follow a slow moving object.
3. Vergence system – eyes move toward or away from either to eliminate diplopia.
4. Vestibular (non-optic) - includes the labyrinthine or otolithic.
5. Position maintenance – maintains eyes on target.

PRIMARY, SECONDARY ACTIONS AND SYNERGISTS OF THE OCULAR MOTOR MUSCLES[1]

Muscle	Primary Action	Secondary Action	Synergists
LR	ABduction	None	SO & I0
MR	ADduction	None	SR & LR
SR	Elevation		IO
		ADduction	MR & IR
		INcycloduction	SO
IR	Depression		SO
		ADduction	MR & SR
		EXcycloduction	IO
SO	INcycloduction		SR
		Depression	IR
		ABduction	LR & IO
IO	EXcycloduction		IR
		Elevation	SR
		Abduction	LR & SO

PRIMARY, SECONDARY ACTIONS AND ANTAGONISTS OF OCULAR MOTOR MUSCLES[1]

Muscle	Action	Antagonists	
		Primary	Secondary
LR	ABduction	MR	SR & IR
MR	ADduction	LR	SO & IO
SR	Elevation	IR	SO
	ADduction		SO, LR, IO
	INcycloduction		IO & IR
IR	Depression	SR	IO
	ADduction		SO, LR, IO
	EXcycloduction		SO, SR
SO	INcycloduction	IO	IR
	Depression		SR & IO
	ABduction		SR, MR, IR
IO	EXcycloduction	SO	SR
	Elevation		IR & SO
	Abduction	MR	SR, IR

EOM Normal Rotations

When all EOM are functioning normally, ocular rotations are considered full, normal eye movements are as follows:

- lateral gaze: able to "bury" sclera.
- up gaze: 3 mm of sclera visible below the iris of each eye.
- down gaze: pupil to lower lid margin.

Innervational Laws

- Sherrington's Law: when agonist contracts the ipsilateral antagonist relaxes an equal amount.
- Hering's Law: when agonist contracts its contralateral synergist (yoke muscle) contracts to an equal amount.

Versions and Greatest Field of Action EOM

- Compare the action of the yoke muscles as the eyes move simultaneously into 2° and 3° positions of gaze.

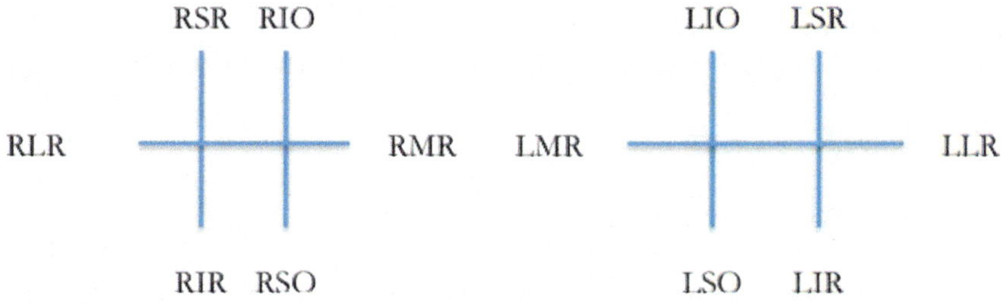

1. Testing Versions
   - Doll's head maneuver in infants
   - Hand puppet or noisemaker in preschool
   - Finger/pen/light in adults

2. Important Points
   - Head must remain in primary position for accuracy.
   - Best to move target horizontally first then up or down to isolate vertical muscles.
   - Graded on -4 to +4 scale (not percentages).
   - Most often looking for under-/over-action of IO or SO muscles.

III. Measurements in Ocular Motility

1. Corneal Light Reflex Test
   Used in patients with:
   - Poor visual acuity/fixation
   - Limited eye movements
   - Poor cooperation
   - *Test is only accurate at near*

2. Hirschberg (H) Test
   - Estimation of misalignment based on light reflex.
   - 1 mm of decentration corresponds to 7 degrees.
   - Penlight held at 1/3 m, and patient asked to fixate on light or target next to it.
   - Important for examiner to be directly in front of patient for accurate measurement.

3. Krimsky (K) Test
   - Same principle as (H), but quantifies deviation with prisms
   - Goal is completely symmetric reflexes
   - Krimsky: prism is placed over the deviating eye.
   - Modified Krimsky: prism is placed over the fixating eye.

4. Single Cover Test

   a) Unilateral tropia
   If *one eye* is constantly deviated and only picks up fixation when the preferred eye is covered and returns to the tropic position when the preferred eye is uncovered, a monocular tropia is present.

   b) Alternate tropia
   If either eye moves to take up fixation when the other eye is covered and maintains fixation when the cover is removed, an alternating tropia is present.

   c) No tropia – phoria
      - If neither eye makes a movement to take up fixation when the other eye is covered because each eye is fixating, no tropia is present.
      - If the eye under cover makes a fusional movement to regain binocular fixation when the cover is removed, the patient has a phoric deviation.

d) Poor vision
If one eye makes wavering or wandering type of movement when the other eye is covered, poor visual acuity should be suspected and the patient may have eccentric (non-foveal) fixation.

5. Alternate prism cover test

a) Comitant (primary and secondary deviation)
Having diagnosed the presence of a heterotropia or heterophoria with the cover-uncover test, the alternate cover test (shifting cover from one eye to the other eye) with prisms is used to quantitate the size of the deviation.

The retino-motor value for each retinal element is determined by the distance of the retinal element from the fovea. Prisms properly placed in front of an eye bring the retinal image closer to the fovea until the correct size prism places the image onto the fovea and the movement is eliminated.

Good clinical technique is important. The examiner must be sure the patient is attending. The prisms are placed:

- Base-out for esodeviation
- Base-in for an exodeviation
- Base-up OD for a left hyper or right hypodeviation
- Base-down OD for a right hyper or left hypodeviation

In other words, the base is placed in the direction the eye moves to take up fixation as it is uncovered. The prisms may be placed in front of either eye or split between the two eyes providing the prisms are placed in the proper direction for each eye. Hold the occluder over each eye long enough so that the patient has sufficient time to take up fixation as you rapidly shift the occluder from one eye to the other. One eye is always covered to maintain constant dissociation. Go to reversal (beyond the end point and movement is now towards the apex of the prism) with prism measurements and subtract 2 prism diopters for the reversal to obtain the full size deviation.

b) Incomitant FOD/FOS (primary and secondary deviation)

When the movement of one eye is reversed, the other eye's movement may not be neutralized. In the presence of a paretic muscle, the angle of deviation is dependent upon which eye fixates. According to Herring's Law of Equal Intervention, the primary deviation is less than the secondary deviation. The primary deviation is with the normal eye fixing (paretic eye deviated) and the secondary deviation is with the paretic eye fixing (the normal eye deviated). The prisms may be placed in front of either eye. During the alternate cover and prism test, the examiner observes and measures only the deviation of the non-fixing eye. To measure the deviation of the left eye with fixing right eye, watch only the left eye's movement until reversals are noted. Then repeat the alternate cover test, observing and measuring the movement of the right eye with OS fixing. If the deviation of the left eye is larger, the fixing right eye has the paretic muscle.

6. Phoria-Tropia-Simultaneous Cover Test

There are cases in which a very small deviation is present with cover-uncover (tropic deviation) which increase with alternate cover (maximal deviation). The maximal deviation minus the tropia is the phoria. In order to measure the size of the tropia from the phoric part of the maximal deviation, the Simultaneous Prism and Cover Test method is used. This is done by placing a prism in front of the deviated eye and simultaneously placing the occluder before the fixing eye. Uncover both eyes and repeat with a larger prism until reversal of deviated eye is observed. The Simultaneous Prism and Cover Test ($S^{\Delta}CT$) is used primarily for micro tropia, monofixational phorias, and phoria-tropias. Basic theory is that peripheral fusion is in effect (phoria) with a facultative central scotoma (tropia).

7. Four Base-Out Prism Test

Purpose

This test is to verify bifoveal fixation or detect a small central scotoma of one eye secondary to a microstrabismus.

Principle

Sudden displacement of an image from the fovea onto parafoveal retina will elicit a refixation movement if the image has been displaced onto normally functioning retina. By Herring's Law of Equal Innervation, both eyes move simultaneously in the same direction (version movement). If a prism is used to suddenly displace an image from the fovea of *one* eye of a patient with normal bifoveal fixation, both eyes will move (version) and then the fellow eye subsequently performs a fusional movement (refixation) in the opposite direction to correct for image displacement from the version. However, if the central foveal and parafoveal area of the *eye behind the prism* is scotomatous (non-functioning), the displacement will not elicit any version or refixation movement. If the central or parafoveal retina of the fellow eye is scotomatous, the version will occur but, the displacement on the fellow eye will not elicit refixation movement.

Procedures

1. Patient has both eyes open (binocular).
2. Patient fixates on an object (attends) during the test.
3. A 4^{Δ} base-out prism is *quickly* placed over the right eye.
4. The examiner observes the movements of the left eye -i.e. normally out and then back in.
5. The test is repeated by' placing the prism over the left eye and observing the right eye.

Responses

1. Scotoma OD (Microtropia)
   a. Prism over OD and no response OU.
   b. Prism over OS and OD moves out (version) but not in (re-fixation).

2. Scotoma OS (Microtropia)
   a. Prism over OD and OS moves out but not in.
   b. Prism over OS and no response OU.

3. Negative (Bifoveal)
   a. Prism over OD and OS goes out and in.
   b. Prism over OS and OD goes out and in.

IV. Sensory and Motor Tests

1. Amplitudes of fusion

   a. Absolute, Relative, Recovery
   Relative fusional amplitudes are the amount of convergence and divergence with accommodation fixed. Blurring is the end point and means accommodation is no longer controlled. For the asthenopic patient, this is more significant than the absolute amplitudes. Absolute amplitudes are the amount of divergence and convergence without controlling accommodation and diplopia is the break point. Recovery point is the point at which the patient regains single binocular vision as the amount of prism is reduced; if lower than 5^{Δ} from the break point, this indicates fatigue in fusional stability.

   b. Clinical Technique
   Clinical testing can be done with a rotary prism, loose prism, or a prism bar and should be done slowly having the patient fix a 20/30 *isolated* letter both at 6 meters and 1/3 meter. Check base-in for divergence and then base-out for convergence.

   c. Norms

   Norms for amplitudes of fusion are:

At Distance		At Near
$6\text{-}7^{\Delta}$	Divergence (Base-In)	$12\text{-}15^{\Delta}$
$25\text{-}35^{\Delta}$	Convergence (Base-Out)	$25\text{-}35^{\Delta}$
$2\text{-}3^{\Delta}$	Vertical (Base-Up and Base-Down	$2\text{-}3^{\Delta}$

2. Near point of convergence

   NPC demonstrates the amount of convergence ability a person can elicit when following an object to his nose.

3. PCB (punctum convergence basalis)

   10 mm from the bridge of the nose to the anterior part of the eye: 15 mm from the anterior part of the cornea to the center of rotation of the eye.

4. Near point of accommodation

   Near point of accommodation (NPA). Clinically, it is the nearest point of clear vision. This measurement should be done separately for each eye and then repeated binocularly. The nearest point at which a small print is readable denotes the NPA. The prince rule or a similar device is used to measure the near point of accommodation in centimeters.

5. Red glass test

   The Red Glass Test is used to diagnose the cortical relationship between the two eyes and the red is a means of differentiating the image of one eye from the image of the other eye. When testing, the red filter is placed before the patient's preferred eye, the patient fixes a white light at 20 feet (later repeated at 13 inches), and the patient is asked how many he sees. The patient may report 1 or 2 images; in order to interpret the response, the examiner must observe whether the patient is phoric or tropic during the testing. The normal sensory for a phoria is fusion and correct diplopia for a tropia. A tropia without diplopia is a sensory adaptation of suppression or ARC ("abnormal fusion"). Incorrect diplopia with tropia denotes ARC.

   Clinically, the examiner must observe whether the patient is phoric or tropic when the patient reports his response. If the patient reports *one* image, the response may mean normal fusion, abnormal binocularity (ARC), or suppression. If the color is both red and white mixed (light red), both eyes are being used. To help the patient distinguish mixed color from red only, cover the unfiltered eye and ask if the color remains the same or becomes darker.

a. Fusion. If the light red (mixed red and white) was claimed, a quick cover-uncover test is performed to see if the patient is phoric. If the cover-uncover test verifies parallelism, the response means normal fusion. If no shift was seen on the cover-uncover test but the patient does not distinguish a color change (darker) when the unfiltered eye is covered, another technique can be used to verify fusion. Move a -1.00 cylinder with the axis at 90° up and down in front of the red filter. The patient should report that the red light appears to move above and below the white if the patient is fusing.

b. ARC. If a light red is claimed and the cover-uncover test reveals a tropia, the patient is reporting abnormal fusion (harmonious ARC).

c. Suppression. If the red does not change when the unfiltered eye is covered and uncovered, the white image was not perceived but suppressed; and the cover-uncover test should reveal a deviation of the unfiltered eye. Suppression may be monocular in which case the patient cannot hold fixation with the non-preferred eye when both eyes are uncovered. Patients with alternate suppression will be able to hold fixation with either eye and switch fixation from the red image to the white image but both images are not seen simultaneously.

   If a patient reports two images *without* alternating eye movements, he is reporting diplopia, which is the normal response to a tropia. In an exotropic patient, the light image falls on the temporal retina of the deviated eye and is perceived in the opposite field producing crossed diplopia. In an esotropic patient, the light image falls on the nasal retina and is seen in the same field producing uncrossed diplopia.

6. Worth-Four-Dot Test

The Worth-Four-Dot Test is used to diagnose the sensorial relationship between the two eyes. Red-green goggles dissociate the images seen by the two eyes. Testing is done with the Worth-Four-Dot flashlight for macular fusion at distance (from 12' to 20') and peripheral fusion at near (13"). If the projector Worth-Four-Dot slide is used for distance, peripheral fusion is being determined.

Fusion ------------------------ 4 dots
2 red and 2 green
1 red and 3 green
1 red and 2 green and 1 mixed

Diplopia ------------------------ 5 dots
2 red and 3 green
crossed or uncrossed

Monocular ------------------------ 2 or 3 dots
Suppression
2 red or 3 green, but only 1 color

Alternate -------------- 2 then 3 dots
Suppression
First one color, then the other color

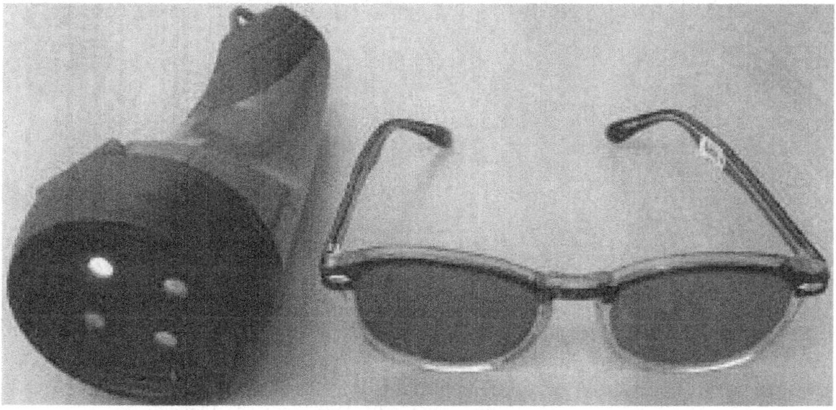

Worth Four Dot Test
Photo courtesy of Kathleen Curtin, University of Michigan

7. Double Maddox Rod Test

This test is a subjective test to determine the presence and quality of a cyclodeviation. Two Maddox Rods are placed at 90°. The red Maddox is placed before the eye that is suspected of having a cyclodeviation and the white Maddox before the other eye. If no vertical is present, a 6^{Δ} vertical prism is placed before one eye to separate the images. The patient fixes a small bright light and is asked if both horizontal lines are parallel.

If both lines are parallel, no cyclodeviation is present. If one line is not perfectly horizontal, the Maddox rod is rotated until both lines are parallel. If the Maddox rod had to be rotated outward to achieve parallelism, an excyclodeviation is present. If the Maddox rod has to be rotated inward to achieve parallelism, an incyclodeviation is present. If torsion is measured to be 5 degrees or greater it becomes a significant problem in strabismus management.

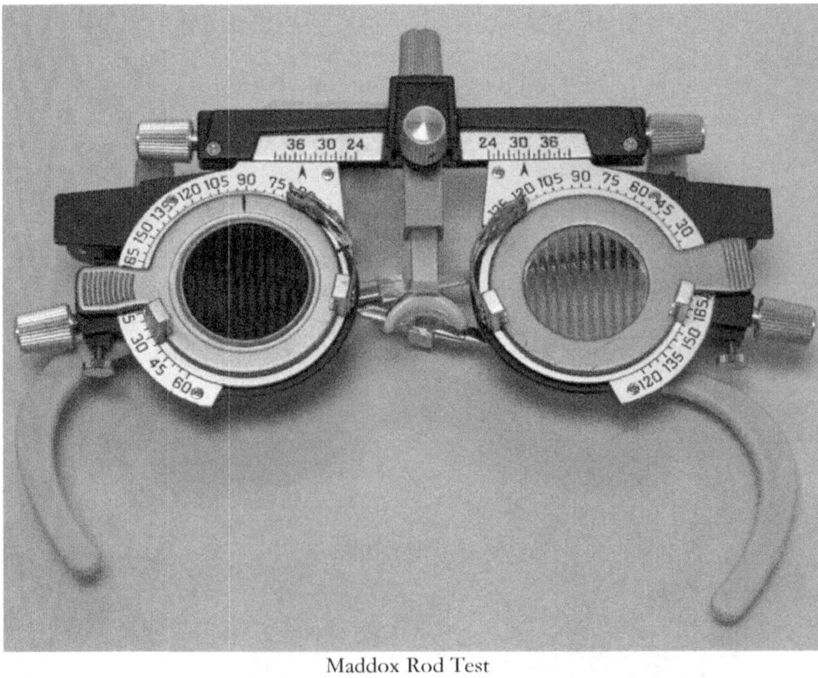

Maddox Rod Test
Photo courtesy of Marc Stephens, University of Michigan

8. Maddox rod test – to evaluate the amount of phoria present.

   The Maddox Rod is composed of a series of cylinders, which produce a linear image of light perpendicular to the direction of cylinders. It is a subjective method in detecting the presence and amount of heterophoria. Horizontal lines are used to measure vertical deviations.

   When testing, the Maddox Rod is placed before the preferred eye and the patient is instructed to fix a small light at 6 meters or 1/3 meter. To prevent the patient's strong impulse to superimpose the light on the line, one eye is occluded and both the light and line are only shown momentarily. The patient is asked the position of the line in relation to the light when both images are seen. If the line is superimposed on the light, the patient is orthophoric. If the line is seen off center, the prisms are placed before one eye until the line is seen passing through the light. The amount of prism required is the size of the phoria deviation.

9. Bagolini Striated Lenses ARC

   Plano lenses have very fine striations etched in them. Placed in a trial frame; one set at 45° and the other at 135° so that the line images are seen obliquely as patient fixes the light. A person with SBV will see a cross passing through the light. ET with NRC X (fixation light above). XT with NRC X (fixation light below). If a person with ET claims a cross at the light X, then the patient must have ARC.

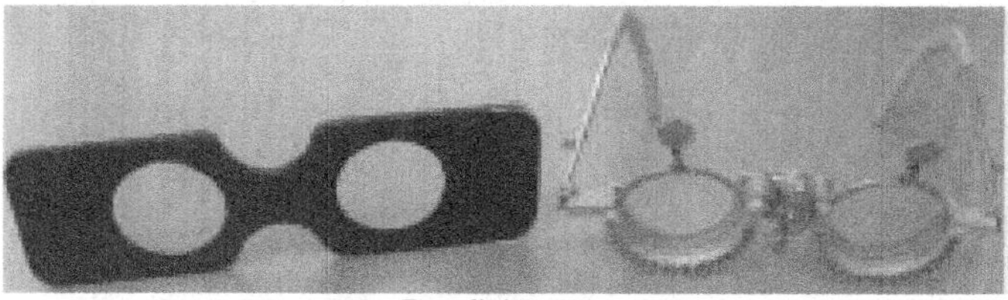

Bagolini Lenses
Photo courtesy of Kathleen Curtin, University of Michigan

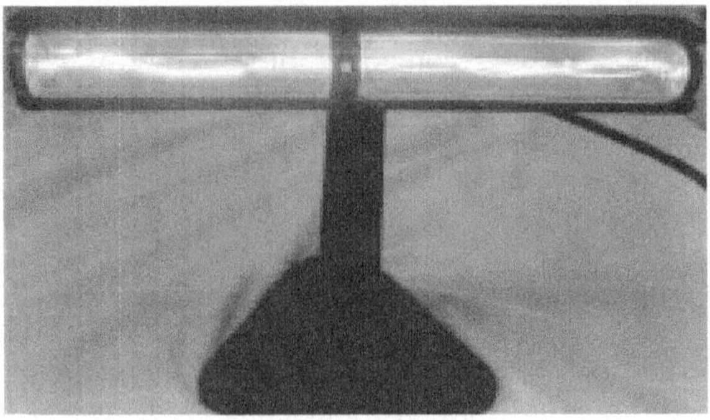

After Image Lamp
Photo courtesy of Kathleen Curtin, University of Michigan

10. After image test ARC

The deviated eye is occluded and the patient is instructed to fix on the dot in the center, while the horizontal filament is shown to the dominant eye for 20 seconds. Light is extinguished, rotated 90°, the opposite is occluded and process repeated. Present the vertical light to the non-dominant eye. Patient is instructed to close their eyes and observe the white lines against the eyelid (positive after image). Patient looks at the blank wall and blinks their eyes to see black lines (negative after image). Each image should have a central gap corresponding to the dot, which indicates the visual direction of the fovea. It is the position of this gap or space in the image that is important. This is a fovea-to-fovea test; it cannot be performed if the patient has eccentric fixation.

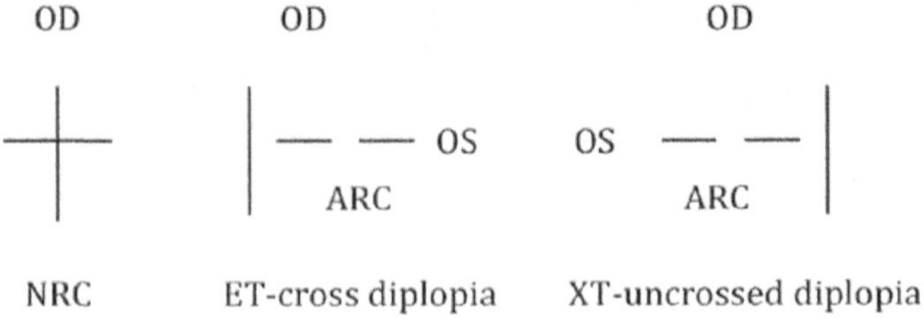

11. Synoptophore (Major Amblyopscope, Troposcope)

This is an instrument that is used in the diagnosis of strabismus and anomalies of binocular vision using visual targets that are presented to each eye through a haploscopic arrangement.

Description of the Synoptophore

It is an instrument that consists of:
- A base with controls.
- 2 tubes with a light source that can be moved horizontally or vertically.
- An illuminated slide carrier and slides with visual targets of various sizes and shapes.
- A reflecting mirror with an eyepiece lens +6.50D. so that the distance for the patient's eye is 15cm. This equals the focal length of the lens so that the eye is focused for distance fixation and the patient does not have to exert any accommodation if he is emmetropic or is wearing his glasses.

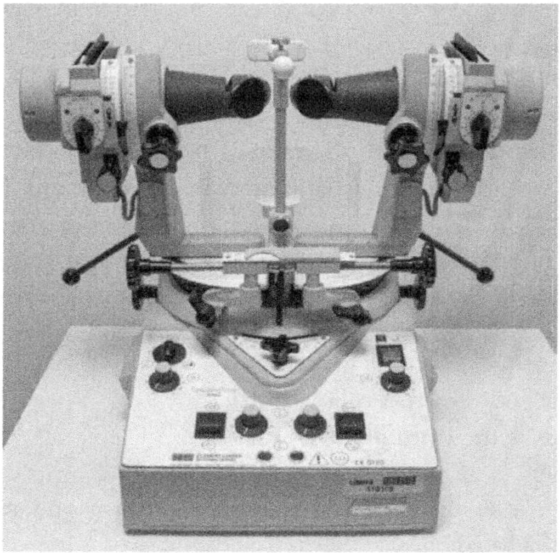

Synoptophore, Clement Clark International Ltd.
Photo courtesy of Marc Stephens, University of Michigan

Disadvantage-proximal convergence is induced.
- There is a mm scale to adjust the IPD.
- A movable chin rest.

The scales measure:

- The horizontal deviation in degrees and prism diopters.
- The vertical deviation in prism diopters.
- The cyclodeviation is measured in degrees.
- Fusional amplitude ranges in degrees and prism diopters – in for convergence and out for divergence.

Slides

- The slides are of various size to test foveal, para foveal, and peripheral function.
- Both slides are placed in the slide holders with the dots facing in the same direction.
- The visual targets test three grades of fusion:

Simultaneous perception slides -(First Degree)

- The slides have a red border.
- The targets are dissimilar.
- This is to test the first grade of fusion that is *sensory fusion.*
- Foveal size targets are the fish and tank.
- Parafoveal - Flowerpot in window.
- Peripheral size - parrot in cage and truck in garage.

Fusion - (Second Degree)

- The slides have a green border.
- They test the second grade of fusion that is *motor fusion.*
- They are similar visual targets with a different detail in each slide.
- Fusion slides are - apple with cherries and a strawberry, a frog on a lily pad with dragonfly and a lily, a bear with blue pants and a red shirt, and a car with a driver and a passenger.

Stereopsis - (Third Degree)

- The slides have a yellow border.
- This is the third grade of fusion.
- They are a circle with lines, a horse and jump with a red and blue flag, a swing with a red and blue flower and fish tank with crab and a lobster.

Special slides

To measure:

- *Torsion* – A circle with a cross slide and the slide with an X surrounded by a border.
- Aniseikonia slides.
- *After image* – the slides have a blue border with a horizontal and vertical lines with a red gap in the middle of the lines.
- *Angle kappa* - the slide has letters and numbers – EDCBA012345 – spaced at 1 degree intervals.

Diagnostic uses

It is used to measure:

- The objective and subjective angles of deviation and the angle anomaly.
- The angle kappa using a special slide on which there are letters and numbers at 1 degree intervals.
- The primary deviation in the deviating eye and fixing with the fixating eye.
- The secondary deviation of the fixating eye and fixing with the deviating eye.
- The deviation in the cardinal directions of gaze.

Estimation of binocular vision:

- The state of retinal correspondence – NRC, ARC, angle of anomaly to determine the type of ARC – harmonious or unharmonious.
- To determine the presence of ARC or NRC there must be a 8 diopter or 4 degree difference between the subjective and objective angle.
- The presence, type and area of suppression – foveal, parafoveal, macular and peripheral.
- Simultaneous perception.
- The presence, degree and range of sensory fusion and motor fusion – fusional divergence and convergence amplitudes – note the break and recovery points.
- The presence of stereopsis.

Clinical application – to determine if surgery is recommended in the presence of cyclotorsion:

- Using the fusion slides, the torsion is corrected and the presence or absence of fusion is determined.
- If fusion is demonstrated then EOM surgery is indicated to correct the torsion and restore fusion.

- If it is absent, this indicates that the patient may not fuse after surgery.

Therapeutic uses in the treatment of:

- Suppression
- ARC
- Eccentric fixation with the Haidinger brushes.
- Accommodative esotropia – dissociation training.
- Improvement of fusional amplitudes.

Method

Diagnostic uses

- The chin rest and the IPD are adjusted.

Measurement of the objective angle of deviation

- The simultaneous perception (SP) slides – the lion and the cage are placed into the slide holders.

To detect the type of deviation a cover test is performed.

- The lion is placed in front of the fixating eye – the right eye - and the cage in front of the left eye and the light in front of the left eye is turned off.
- The right arm is set at zero and the left one in the vicinity of zero – on the base outside for esodeviations and base in for exodeviations.

To measure the deviation an alternate cover test is performed.

- With the patient fixating the lion with the right eye, the light in front of the left eye is turned on as the light in front of the right eye is turned off.
- The patient is asked to look directly in the center of the cage and watch the left eye as it moves to take up fixation.
- The left arm is moved
    - in toward a convergent position - if the eye is seen to move out = ET.
    - out for a divergent position = XT.
    - If the eye moves downward the tube has to be raised = HT
    - If it moves upwards the tube is lowered = hypotropia.
- The alternating flashing is continued until there is no movement when either eye picks up fixation.
- The reading on the left arm on the horizontal scale and the vertical scale represents the objective angle of deviation.

- For example if the left arm is at base out 15 pd and has to be raised by 2 pd then the angle is recorded as ET 15, LHT 2.

Measurement of the subjective angle of deviation

- If the lion is in the cage, then superimposition is present and the objective angle is also the subjective angle.
- If this is not the case, the patient is asked to move the left arm until the lion is in the cage. This is the patient's subjective angle.
- In some cases the lion may not be placed in the cage and is seen to suddenly cross to the other side of the cage – crossed diplopia in ET, or uncrossed diplopia with XT. The crossing point is the subjective angle.
- Suppression may also be present.

Measurement of the angle of anomaly

- The difference between the objective and subjective angle is the angle of anomaly.
- If the objective angle is ET 20 base out and the subjective angle is 6 base out, the angle of anomaly is 14 pd.

Measurement of the angle of deviation at near

- *-3.00 spheres* are inserted into the lens holders in front of the eye piece lenses.
- The patient has to exert 3.00D of accommodation in order to get a clear image of the slides.
- Each eye exerts 3pd of convergence for each diopter of accommodation. C = 3pd/A=1D.
- Or 9pd of convergence on one eye. +3.00 lens = 3D x 3 A = 9pd of C for one eye or 18 pd for both eyes – 9+9 = 18 pd
- IPD = 60mm. (for a smaller IPD the convergence requirement is less, a bigger one – more).
- To record the angle of deviation, either 18 pd is added in an ET or subtracted for an XT from the readings.
- If a recording of 20 base out is recorded as ET 2, 20pd – 18pd = 2 pd.
- 20 pd base as XT 38 pd. 20pd + 18 pd = 38 pd.

Measurement of subjective cyclodeviations

- SP slides are used – the lion in front of the right eye and the cage in front of the left eye.
- The patient is asked to look at each one in turn and is asked if the cage appears level.

- If it is tilted – torsion is present.
- If the left side of the cage is lower than the right – intorsion is present and extorsion if it is lower on the left side.
- The tilt is corrected and read in degrees on the torsion scale that is located on the slide holder.
- The images are tilted in the opposite direction to the tilt of the eye.

Determining angle kappa

- A special slide that consists of a row of number and letters (EDCBA012345) at 1 degree intervals.
- The patient is asked to look at the zero.
- *Positive angle kappa* - The corneal light reflex is on the nasal side of the pupil, appears XT.
- *Negative angle kappa* - The corneal light reflex is on the temporal side of the pupil, appears ET.
- The patient is asked to look in turn at either the letters or numbers until the reflex is centered.
- The degree of deviation corresponding to the letter or number is recorded.
- For example – if the corneal reflex in the right eye is centered on the C, the patient has a 3 degree negative angle kappa in the right eye.

Determining fusional amplitudes

- The fusion slides (green border) are placed into the slide holders.
- These are similar targets with control marks for each eye – mouse/bear with red shirt and blue pants.)
- If the patient fuses the targets and sees them as one with both control marks, the arms are locked at the objective angle, divided equally between the two arms.
- Using the horizontal controls both arms are first diverged and the point where fusion breaks is recorded.
- The arms are then moved back to a less divergent position and the point at which fusion is recovered is recorded.
- The arms continue to be converged until fusion breaks and is recovered.

Stereopsis

- The stereo slides (yellow border) are placed in the slide holders.
- The image should be seen as a single image with both the controls.
- The target is seen in depth – the swing appears towards or away from you.

Recording results

Distance:

Objective and subjective angle – ET 26, RHT 2.
First and second grade fusion – present at angle.
Convergence – to BO 40/recovery at BO 30.
Stereopsis – present with foveal, para foveal or peripheral slides.

Near with -3.00D spheres:

Objective and subjective angles – ET 46, RHT 2.
Convergence – to BO 58/recovery at BO 46.
Divergence – no divergence past angle, suppression OD.
Stereopsis – absent.

12. Lancaster Red Green Test

The Lancaster Red-Green is a *foveal projection* test used for detecting incomitance of a deviation in a patient with normal sensory relationship. It is not reliable in patients with ARC and deep suppression.

The tangent screen is composed of lines which form squares 7 cm apart. The patient is positioned 1 or 2 meters from the tangent screen and the eyes should be at the level with the *zero* center mark on the screen. At 2 meters, each square subtends an angle of 3.5^{o} or 7^{Δ} for 1 meter. The patient is given red and green goggles (usually red in front of OD, green OS) and a torch flashlight is held by the patient and the other held by the examiner. One torch flashlight projects red which can only be seen through the red lens and the other torch flashlight projects green which can be seen only through the green lens. The color held by the examiner *determines the fixing eye.* For example, the examiner projects a green light on the zero mark and the patient is asked to superimpose his red light on the examiner's green light. This is repeated in the 6 diagnostic positions of gaze. The distance of light (projected by the patient) from the diagnostic positions (projected by the examiner) determines the amount of deviation. The flashlights are traded and the test is repeated. The results are plotted on a chart that is an exact duplicate of the screen. Once plotted one can easily observe 1) the diagnostic position at which the separation of light is greatest, 2) primary and secondary deviation, 3) identify the paretic muscles.

Chapter 2

FORMS OF RETINAL CORRESPONDENCE

NRC – Normal Retinal Correspondence
(Corresponding Retinal Elements)

ARC – Anomalous Retinal Correspondence
(Noncorresponding Retinal Elements)

I. Introduction – Horopter & Types of ARC

A. Physiological Factors[2]

Localization is based on physiological factors. *Objective* aspect is the correct geometric localization of an object in space. The objective line of direction (visual axis) is the line drawn from the fixation object through space and the optical system of the eye to the retina. Normally, light from an object located directly ahead stimulates the fovea.

A *retinal element* refers to a rod or cone together with all the chain of cells connecting that sensory cell with the occipital visual cortex.

Subjective aspect (projection) is the place in space where an object *appears* to be situated which depends on the spatial value of the *particular retinal element stimulated.* Each retinal element has its own particular direction in which it localizes objects that stimulate it, which is the visual *direction* of that retinal element. The fovea normally has a zero value visual direction.

The objective line of direction visual axis and the *subjective visual direction* normally coincide.

For every point on the retina of one eye there is a point on the retina of the other eye which is stimulated by the same object. Retinal elements in each eye, which normally are stimulated by the same object, are called *normal retinal corresponding elements.* These are corresponding retinal elements that have the same visual direction. The foveas are corresponding points "par excellence".

An object stimulating non-corresponding retinal points is seen double because each point has a different visual direction. Slightly disparate retinal elements are fused if the retinal elements are within *Panum's fusional* area and result in stereopsis instead of diplopia. The amount of disparity fused is very small near the fovea but increases in size as the peripheral retinal areas are stimulated.

B. Horopter

Locus of points in a space which at a given distance simultaneously stimulate corresponding retinal elements therefore giving rise to a single image.

Empiric horopter forms a variable line depending on the distance of fixation object from the eye:

1. Fixation object 2 meters away - horopter is a straight line passing through the fixation point.
2. Fixation object nearer than 2 meters – horopter is curved, concave to the face.
3. Fixation object is beyond 2 meters – horopter is curved, concave to the face.

Images falling on non-corresponding points (each having different visual direction) are seen double. However, slightly disparate retinal points to be stimulated by similar images produce a single image because the retina points fall within Panum's area (stereopsis).

Representative of Panum's fusional space.

Fixation distance 1 METER –
horizontal meridian for the horopter (YY) one meter away.

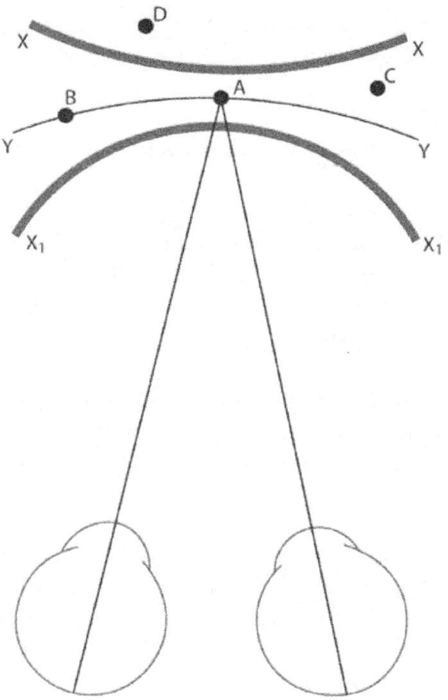

{Y Y} Horizontal meridian for the Horopter 1 meter away

{XX_1, XX} Limits of Panum's fusional areas in the retina in relation to the horopter

A- The fixation point.
B- On the horopter - imaged on corresponding retinal points seen as one.
C- Is off the horopter but within Panum's fusional areas - imaged on non-corresponding points but is seen with depth effect (stereopsis) and *not double.*
D- Is off the horopter and outside Panum's fusional area – imaged on non-corresponding points seen double (physiologic diplopia).

Panum found that in the region near the fovea only a *slight degree* of disparity was possible before stereopsis failed and diplopia occurs; nearer to the periphery, more widely disparate retinal points give rise to stereopsis rather than diplopia.

Therefore, imaging areas of disparate points are very small near the fovea and increase in size as they approach the periphery of the retina.

Panum's area – Fusional area around corresponding points *in the retina.*

Panum's space: The space on either side of the horopter containing objects in space, images of which will fall on slightly disparate retinal elements within Panum's fusional areas of the two retinas so that they are found as stereopsis.

Anomalous retinal correspondence is an attempt of the strabismic patient to obtain some semblance of normal binocular vision. It is a binocular phenomenon though monocularly either eye picks up fixations with the fovea.

In heterotropic patients non-corresponding retinal elements outside of Panum's fusional area are stimulated. Normal localization of the deviated eye results in diplopia rather than fusion. Anomalous localization allows an 'extra foveal' element of the deviating eye to acquire a correspondence with the fovea of the fixing eye. In heterotropia-anomalous, retinal correspondence may develop for the purpose of eliminating diplopia (and confusion) and regaining a semblance of binocularity with some form of stereopsis. It is a binocular phenomenon, though monocularly either eye picks up fixation with the fovea.

C. Two types of ARC

Harmonious ARC	Unharmonious ARC
30 $^{\Delta}$ Esotropia	30 $^{\Delta}$ Esotropia – Objective Angle 20 $^{\Delta}$ Esotropia – Subjective Angle

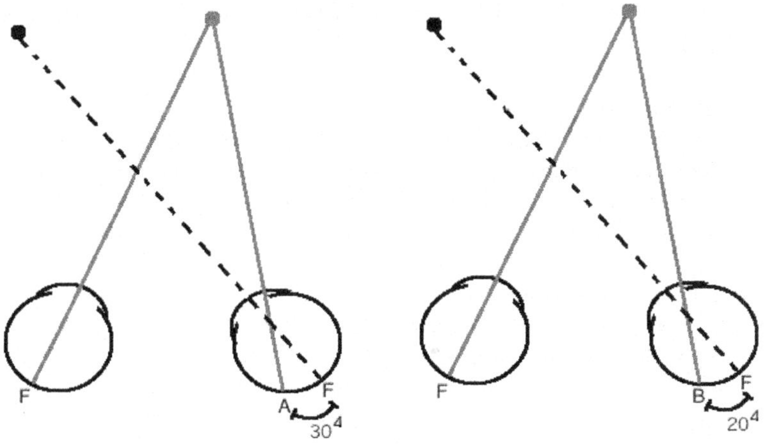

Angle of anomaly is equal to the angle of strabismus	Angle of anomaly is not equal to the angle of strabismus

1. Harmonious ARC

Angle of anomaly is equal to the angle of strabismus and therefore the subjective angle is zero. In harmonious ARC a retinal element in the deviated eye which is at the *exact point* (A) *where the image falls* or the deviating eye *acquires* correspondence with the fovea of the fixing eye.

2. Unharmonious ARC

The subjective angle is not equal to the objective angle of strabismus. The subjective angle is greater than zero but less than the objective angle of strabismus. The fovea of the fixing eye acquires a correspondence with external stimuli of the deviated eye but not at the exact objective angle of deviation (as in harmonious ARC). The pseudo fovea is at a point (B) *less* than the objective angle of deviation. The patient with unharmonious ARC has learned to use their eyes at a less crossed angle in an attempt toward binocularity.

NOTE: Some do not believe unharmonious ARC exists but it is demonstrated on a variety of tests. It has been explained that it could be due to the patient having a change in angle of strabismus and the sensory adjustment hasn't had time to 'catch up' with the change in angle of strabismus. Bagolini has never been able to demonstrate unharmonious ARC with the striated lens following surgical correction and this definitely demonstrates a rapid sensory adjustment. He feels that it exists because of the methods used in testing.

D. Terminology

Clinically, we speak of the *objective angle* as the amount of deviation measured by the examiner and neutralized so that the image of the fixation object falls on the fovea of each eye, such as the alternate cover and prism test or alternate cover test on the amblyoscope.

Subjective angle is the amount of correction in prism diopters in which the patient informs the examiner that he can superimpose and fuse the images of the test object.

Angle of anomaly is the difference of the objective angle minus the subjective angle. In normal retinal correspondence the objective angle and subjective angle are the same, Therefore, the angle of anomaly is zero. In unharmonious ARC, the objective angle does not equal the subjective angle. The subjective angle is less than the objective angle; the angle of anomaly is not zero. In harmonious ARC, the subjective angle is equal to the objective angle.

In summary:

Objective test – depends upon findings of the examiner – independent of patient's response.

Subjective test – depends upon a patient's response.

Subjective angle – The angle on the synoptophore at which the patient can superimpose test object slides is different from the objective angle which shows ARC (at least 8^{Δ} or 4° difference to demonstrate ARC).

Objective angle – The angle to which examiner manipulates the arms of the synoptophore so that the image of test object slides fall on the fovea of each eye.

E. Definitions

Anomalous retinal correspondence can be defined in more than one way.

1. ARC is present when two foveae no longer have a common visual direction.

2. ARC is a binocular condition where the fovea of the fixing eye is used in conjunction with a point other than the fovea of the deviating eye.

3. ARC is a binocular condition where the angles of deviation measured objectively and subjectively are not coincident. The difference between the two angles is known as the angle of anomaly.

4. ARC is a binocular condition where there has been a rearrangement of the normally common visual directions of the retinal elements of the two eyes. Corresponding retinal elements lose their common visual direction while disparate retinal elements acquire a common visual direction.

F. Prognosis for ARC to Develop

Anomalous retinal correspondence is more likely to develop in small to moderate degree manifest deviations with a relatively constant long-standing and stable angle. In large angles of deviation, there is little reward for development of ARC because the peripheral retina has very low visual attention. It is seldom present in accommodative strabismus, intermittent strabismus, and incomitant deviations due to variability of the angle of deviation. It is rare in alternating strabismus.

Cases in which ARC is more likely to develop:

1. Moderate degree of ET (esotropia) and relatively stable angle of deviation.

2. In small angles of deviation under 10 prism diopters the image may fall within Panum's fusional area.

II. Sensory Tests for ARC

Clinical tests are based on two principles: (1) to assess visual direction of the two foveae, and (2) to compare the subjective localization of images with the objective angle of deviation.

A. Diplopia Test - Method I

1. Red filter over preferred eye. Patient fixes on distant or near light.
2. Place vertical prism (10^{Δ} BU or BD) in front of one eye to help overcome suppression.

Results: If red light is seen above white light in presence of 30^{Δ} ET, this indicates harmonious ARC.

B. Diplopia Test - Method II

1. Objective angle is neutralized with appropriate prisms and checked by cover test.

2. Red filter is placed in front of one eye. Check again if deviation is still neutralized, then ask patient if images are superimposed. If images are not seen superimposed, reduce prisms until the images are seen superimposed or change from crossed to uncrossed or vice versa. If more than 8^{Δ} difference from objective angle, ARC is present.

C. Bagolini Striated Lens

Plano lenses have very fine striations etched in them. They are placed in a trial frame; one is set at 45° and the other at 135° so that the line images are seen obliquely as the patient fixes a light. A person with single binocular vision will see a cross passing through the light. ET with NRC  (fixation light above), XT with NRC  (fixation light below).

If a person with an ET claims a cross at the light  then they must have ARC. If only one line is seen passing through the light, suppression of one eye is indicated.

NOTE: The Bagolini lens has the same effect as the Maddox Rod but does not dissociate the eyes by presenting an obstacle to vision and it reduces the artificiality of the testing situation. It represents the most 'normal' seeing conditions.

D. Bielschowsky After Image Test

One eye is occluded and the patient is instructed to fix a dot in the center of a horizontal filament of light for approximately 20 seconds. The light is then extinguished, rotated to 90°, the other eye occluded, and the process is repeated. Present the horizontal light first to the normally dominant eye and then the vertical light to the non-dominate eye.

Results: The patient is instructed to close their eyes and observe the white lines against his eyelids and draw the arrangement of lights seen (the positive after image). Then the patient looks at a blank wall, blinks their eyes, and observes the position of the black lines seen against the wall (negative after image). Each image should have a central gap corresponding to the dot which indicates the visual direction of the fovea. It is the position of this gap or space in the image which is important.

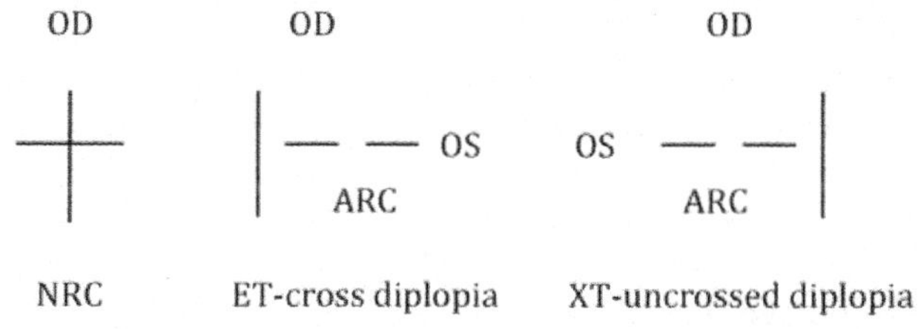

TIP: The distance between the gaps is determined by the angle of anomaly and not the angle of deviation; gaps show directional value of foveas.

IMPORTANT: If ARC is revealed on this test, it is well established. It is possible to show NRC on this test and ARC on other tests because the after image test makes no attempt to produce normal conditions of seeing and is more likely to reveal the original (normal) correspondence.

Disadvantages

a. Difficult to use with uncooperative patients because of the necessity of accurate observations.
b. Does not necessarily diagnose what the patient is doing under every day conditions.
c. Complete suppression of one image may occur.

E. Major Amblyoscope (Synoptophore)

Patient is asked to move the arm of the troposcope before the non-fixing eye until they see the images superimposed or until they see them cross from side to side. The subjective angle at which this occurs is compared to the objective angle of deviation. The angle of anomaly should not be less than 8 prism diopters because it can be confused with:

1. Suppression - Small area of dense central suppression simulating an angle of an anomaly.
2. Accommodation - angle of deviation may vary on dissociation.
3. Small degree of incomitance - apparent angle of anomaly as patient changes fixation from one eye to the other.

IMPORTANT: Degree to which ARC is established can be assessed using different size 1° and 2° slides.

Each eye is covered in turn and the patient is asked to note any movement of the fixation object. The object should move to a degree corresponding to the angle of deviation if NRC is present. If no movement is observed, suspect ARC.

III. Objective Tests

Press-on prisms are a useful tool to assess patient response to surgery.

When patients cannot reliably respond to sensory tests, the prism adaptation test (PAT) may help to prognosticate surgical outcome. Press-on prisms are given in an amount to slightly overcorrect the deviation and are placed completely in front of the preferred eye in children, non-preferred eye in adult, or equally in front of both eyes. If after one to two weeks wearing the prism the patient returns to his original deviation, this informs the surgeon to be more aggressive in the surgical procedure.

IV. Treatment of ARC Patients

A. General Management

Occlusion to eliminate amblyopia or alternate occlusion to prevent reinforcement of ARC which is a binocular phenomenon before surgical management.

B. Cosmetically Acceptable Patients

If patient has a small angle deviation (10-20$^{\Delta}$), VA is fairly equal, gross fusion and gross stereopsis, no treatment is given in an attempt to break ARC. In fact, some authorities advocate reinforcing and firmly establishing the ARC in order to give a more refined and stable form of binocular vision. The method of treatment used in firmly establishing the ARC is mainly with the amblyoscope. Have the arms set at the patient's subjective angle and increase divergence and convergence amplitudes from the subjective angle.

IMPORTANT: The majority of patients in this group are given no treatment and are just observed at 6 month intervals to check if ARC pattern is firmly maintained.

C. Orthoptic Management

1. Occlusion - to equalize VA and then alternate occlusion continued preoperatively to prevent reinforcement of ARC.

2. If orthoptic treatment is considered, the orthoptic methods performed on the Synoptophore are as follows:

   a. Bi-retinal kinetic stimulation
   The major amblyoscope tubes are locked at the patient's objective angle and the patient is instructed to fix straight ahead into the distance through the pictures. The tubes are then moved back and forth sideways to stimulate retinal corresponding points. The patient must not watch the pictures.

   b. Massage of the macular area
   The major amblyoscope tubes are set at the patient's objective angle and the patient is instructed to fix steadily on the target

before the fixing eye. The other tube is moved from side to side over the objective angle while the patient tries to see that target crossing backwards and forwards over the fixation object.

c. Mayou Technique
A foveal target is presented to the non-dominant eye and boxes of varying size to the fixing eye. Starting with the largest box, the patient is asked to move the tube from side to side over the target. This may cover a large area at first, the area gradually decreasing. When the images can be seen superimposed, smaller boxes are used until foveal targets can be superimposed without movement.

d. Flashing
The major amblyoscope tubes are locked at the objective angle and large, bright targets are used. The illumination is increased to maximum before the non-dominant eye. Alternate flashing is then carried out and the patient attempts to see the images come closer and eventually superimpose.

All exercises are objective and can be dull for the patient. Many patients may eventually give correct answers merely because they are bored.

D. Surgery

Aim is placing the visual axis parallel in order to facilitate constant bifoveal stimulation. Since patients with ARC have an intense motivation to return to their anomalous angle, the surgery considered is usually more aggressive than in patients with NRC.

Chapter 3

DIPLOPIA

I. Binocular Diplopia

Two images seen of one object -- non-corresponding *retinal* elements being stimulated.

Fixation object stimulates the fovea of fixing eye and a point other than the fovea in the deviating eye and therefore is seen *double*. The two retinal points stimulated do not have the same visual direction.

Right Esotropia

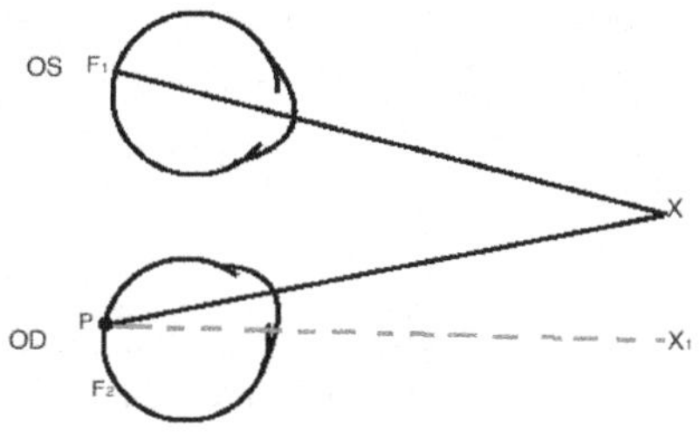

F_1 & F_2 = Fovea
X = Fixation object
X_1 = Second image, homonymous diplopia seen by P (nasal retinal point) in deviated eye.

Right Exotropia

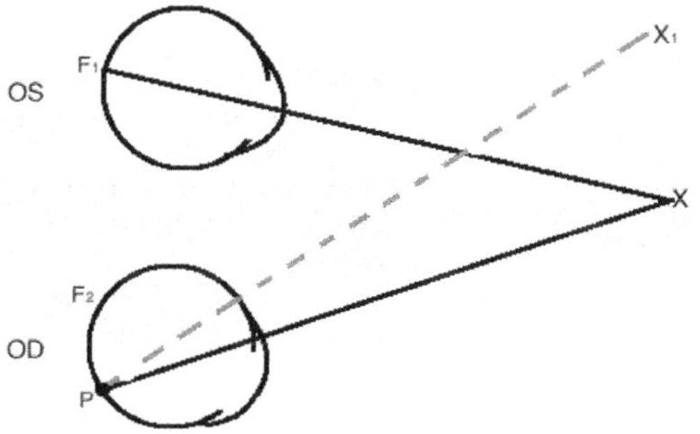

F_1 & F_2 = Fovea
X = Fixation object
X_1 = Second image, heteronymous diplopia seen by P (temporal retinal point) in deviated eye.

Right Hypertropia

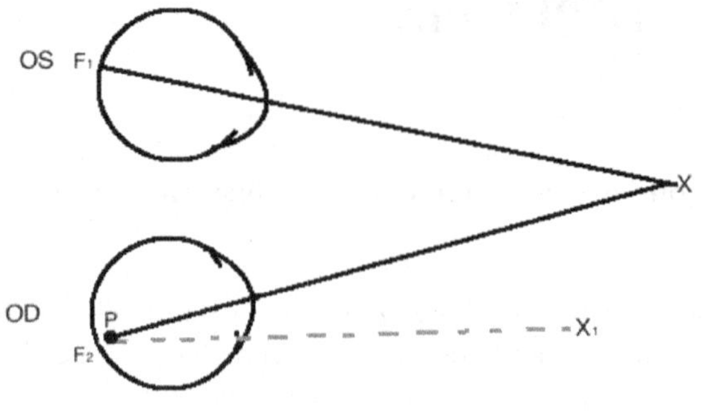

F_1 & F_2 = Fovea
X = Fixation object
X_1 = Second image, seen by P (superior retinal point) in deviated eye and projected inferiorly.

II. Physiological Diplopia

Objects *situated* nearer than the fixation object or *beyond* the fixation object are falling or *non-corresponding retinal* elements and seen double.

1. Homonymous or uncrossed diplopia

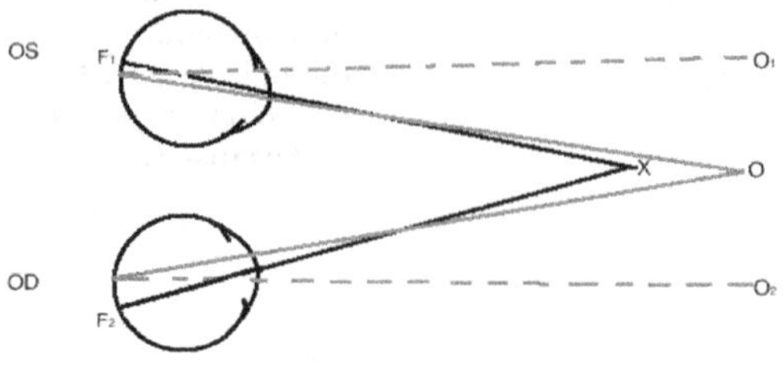

F_1 & F_2 = Fovea
X = Near fixation object
O = Distance object stimulating nasal retina points and being projected temporally.
O_1 & O_2 = Homonymous physiological diplopia

2. Heteronymous or crossed diplopia

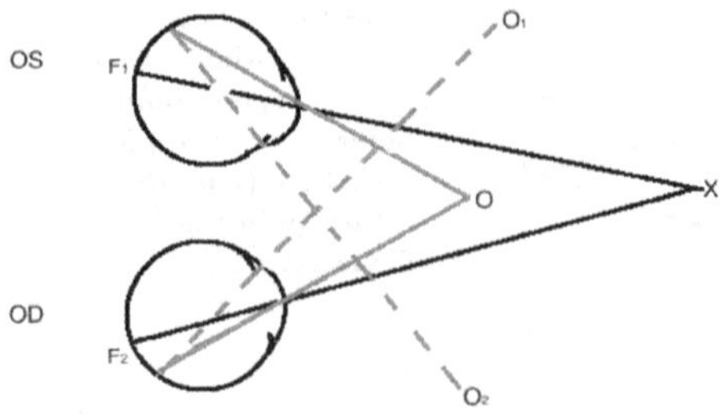

F_1 & F_2 = Fovea
X = Distance fixation object
O = Near object stimulating temporal retinal points and being projected nasally
O_1 & O_2 = Heteronymous physiological diplopia

In physiological diplopia we are normally *conscious* and can easily be aware of it (Teach method). This phenomenon is used in treatment of *heterophoria.*

III. Pathological Diplopia

Onset of manifest deviation - diplopia or confusion may occur.

Confusion is a condition in *which dissimilar objects stimulate* both foveas and are *projected* to the same position in space. This is *caused* by each fovea having the same visual direction.

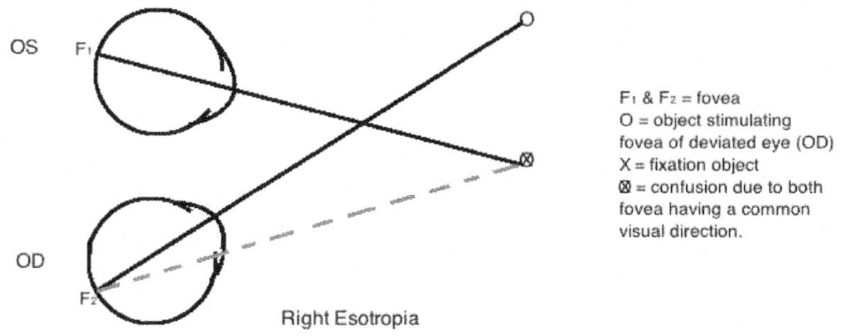

IV. Uniocular Diplopia

Two images seen from one eye.

A. Pathological uniocular diplopia

1. *Large* displacement of images.
   a. Dry eyes
   b. Displacement of lens
   c. Two pupils or coloboma of iris
   d. Retinal detachment – involving the macula
      Maculopathy
      sub-retinal neovascular membrane
      macular epiretinal membrane

2. *Small* displacement of images – one image behind the other.
   a. Uncorrected astigmatism
   b. Lens opacities
   c. Air bubbles in the aqueous or vitreous

B. Physiological uniocular diplopia. Patient may complain of seeing two images of one object during treatment of ARC or on the major amblyoscope. Because of dual projection of a retinal point, abnormal projection co-exists before ARC is overcome.

V. Paradoxical Diplopia

Heteronymous diplopia *occurring* post-operatively where the visual axes are now parallel but the fovea continues to project abnormally.

ARC *must have existed* pre-operatively.

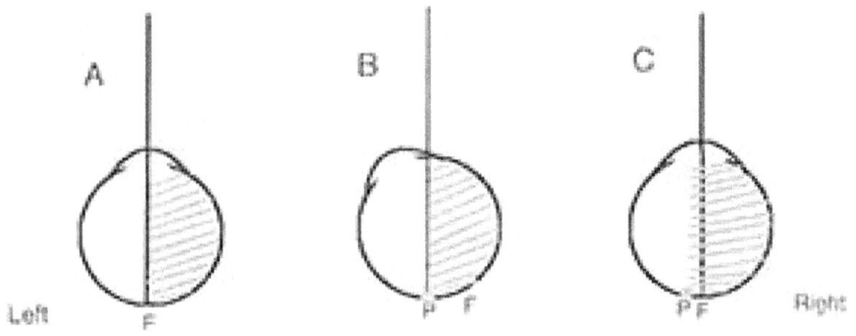

A. Represents a normal right eye – darker area represents the nasal visual field and the light area represents the temporal visual field.

B. Represents a patient with a right esotropia and an abnormal retinal correspondence. The darker area to P represents the nasal visual field – the lighter area represents to temporal visual field.

C. Represents "B" after the eye has been straightened by surgery. The area PF continues to represent nasal visual field resulting in crossed diplopia where in normal correspondence there would be uncrossed diplopia – a paradox.

Chapter 4

AMBLYOPIA

Evaluation and Treatment

I. Introduction

A. Definition

Diminution of VA of one eye with a difference of one or more lines on the vision chart while wearing any significant optical correction. If there is no *organic* cause, it is a functional amblyopia.

B. Classification (Von Noorden)[3]

1. *Strabismic amblyopia*
   Defect of visual acuity in one eye without visible pathologic changes in the fundus or refractive media. It is found in patients with strabismus or a history of such imbalance. It is a result of longstanding active inhibition of macular function of form vision in the course of an adaptation to avoid visual confusion or diplopia.

2. *Ametropic / Anisometropic Amblyopia*
   Impaired vision due to uncorrected refractive error or a high degree of anisometropia.

3. *Organic amblyopia* (sensory amblyopia)
   Although the fundus appears normal, anatomic damage to the retina or visual pathway must be assumed to be present. Example: possible retinal hemorrhage in the newborn infant that then clears with a visible trace of macular impairment. Example: corneal and lens opacities.

   IMPORTANT: Neutral density filter placed in front of the amblyopic eye will differentiate between organic or functional amblyopia.

   Functional – Visual acuity remains the same or improved
   Organic – Visual acuity is decreased

C. Risk factors for amblyopia

Anisometropia
(spherical or cylinder) > 1.5 D
Any manifest strabismus 23% improve with full time spectacle correction

{ Hyperopia > 3.5 D in any meridian
Myopia > 3.0 D in any meridian }

Astigmatism > 1.0 D
Ptosis < 1 mm margin reflex distance
VA → per age appropriate standard

VA Per Age

AGE	VA
4 months	20/2000
6 months	20/1000
9 months	20/200
1 year	20/150
2 years	20/45
3 years	20/30
4 years	20/25
5 years	20/20

D. Testing vision

Vision should be tested whole line letters (cortical VA) as well as isolated letters (angular VA) due to the crowding phenomenon in amblyopia. It is very important to test near VA. If near VA is better than distance vision it indicates excellent potential for improvement with treatment. Refer to vision assessment in preverbal and verbal children in Basic Tests Chapter One.

E. Amblyopia with Central Fixation and Eccentric Fixation

1. Central Fixation

The fovea is the carrier of the principal visual direction with a retinal motor values at zero. When the preferred eye is occluded, the amblyopic eye picks up fixation with the fovea. This indicates excellent potential for normal VA.

2. Eccentric Fixation

A retinal element other than the fovea becomes the carrier of the principle visual direction. When the preferred eye is occluded, the amblyopic eye does not pick up fixation with true fovea. In other words, an eccentric retinal element has assumed all the characteristic of the fovea except potential of normal VA. In eccentric fixation, the patient has separation difficulty when whole letters are presented. When linear VA is markedly reduced compared to isolated letters, eccentric fixation is probably present.

F. Testing Fixation

1. Visuscope to Diagnose the Presence of Central or Eccentric Fixation

The visuscope is a conventional ophthalmoscope in which a small star is projected onto the fundus and the patient is asked to fixate on the star. If the foveal reflex is seen on the center of the projected star (☆), the patient's fixation is central. If the star does not fall on the foveal reflex, the following types of eccentric fixation may be observed.

a. Types of Eccentric Fixation

1. Central but unsteady (i.e. fixation shifts on and off the fovea).

2. Fixates a point close to the fovea, either nasal, temporal, superior or inferior. The distance can be measured by projecting a disc that has several rings surrounding the star. Each ring is equal to ½ degree and the location of the fovea on the rings determines the amount of eccentricity. When the fixation point is to the nasal side of the disc, it is called Ceco Central.

3. No definite fixation point (patient's fixation constantly wavers) indicates a very poor prognosis because the patient is unable to establish a definite pattern.

b. Technique for visuscope or ophthalmoscope examination

Examine the dominant fixing eye first and cover the eye not under examination. Use low illumination to prevent dazzling of the retina. First look with the green filter disc before switching to the white light when assessing the area of the retina. This can be performed with an ophthalmoscope by displaying the disc with the circles and instruct the patient to fix in the center of the smaller circle to check fixation pattern.

2. Haidinger Brushes to Diagnose Central or Eccentric Fixation

   The Koordinator or ocular synoptophore are instruments that contain the Haidinger Brushes. Only the macular and paramacular areas can perceive the Haidinger Brush. It is produced by a rotating Polaroid, cobalt lens which stimulates the macular-papillar bundles and the propeller-like image observed is the Haidinger Brush. A circular aperture (measured in degrees) is placed in front of the lens containing the Haidinger Brush. As the field is slowly diminished with the circular aperture, the patient will inform the examiner when the Haidinger Brush disappears. *If central*, the patient is aware of the Haidinger Brush with the smallest aperture opening of ½ centimeter. *If eccentric*, the Haidinger Brush will disappear as the field is diminished, depending upon the degree of eccentricity. If the eccentricity is outside the macular area, the patient will not be aware of the Haidinger Brush.

   NOTE: The Haidinger Brush phenomenon is not only used in evaluation but also in pleoptic treatment.

3. Past Pointing

   Small dots of various sizes are drawn on a white sheet of paper and the patient is given a pointer with a sharp tip. With his dominant eye occluded, the patient is told to point directly to the dots. This can also be done with the amblyopic eye occluded to check the comparison of either eye fixing. If the patient is central, he will point directly on the dot. If eccentric, he will point to the side of the dot. This is based on the concept that, in the absence of foveal fixation, the patient does not have a true sense of spatial value.

II. Amblyopia Treatment in Patients Through Three Years of Age With Central or Eccentric Fixation

(Significant refraction error should be prescribed)

Full-time skin patch of the dominant eye during waking hours but patch should be removed at bedtime. If a significant refractive error is present, correction should be given. In children age three or younger with central fixation will improve very quickly; those with eccentric fixation will improve at a slower rate but prognosis is excellent because the eccentricity is not firmly established.

Infants below 1 year of age should be checked weekly to guard against the dominant eye becoming amblyopic. Children from age one through three years should be seen at two week intervals. Once the patient can fix steadily and voluntarily with the amblyopic eye, begin to alternate patch three hours a day. At the next visit (2-3 weeks), the patient should be able to alternate freely and be ready to be treated for the strabismic problem. Patients that have marked anisometropia (central or eccentric) have good prognosis in the age group.

NOTE: According to the PEDIG Study – four to six hours of occlusion should be sufficient to eliminate amblyopia in this age group.

III. Amblyopia Treatment Ages Four to Twelve Years with Central Fixation

In visual acuity ranging from 20/80 → 20/200 or more initiate full time skin patch of the dominant eye. Patch is removed at bedtime and immediately applied in the morning. In older children, if the patch cannot be accepted during school hours, patch is worn after school and full time on weekends. Improvement is slower, normal acuity should be obtained.

During occlusion of the dominant eye, the child is encouraged to sit back from TV, and do various detailed near work (i.e. drawing, tracing, models, reading, stitchery). Total skin occlusion of the dominant eye is continued until 20/50 VA is obtained. Patients are seen at three to four week intervals for VA check.

Once 20/50 VA is achieved, discontinue the skin patch and initiate Bangerter foil full time in front of preferred eye usually 0.3 foil. Translucent (magic transparent) scotch tape or clear contact paper five hours a day on the lens in front of the preferred eye can be an alternate method of treatment.

When the vision in the amblyopic eye is equal to the vision of the dominant eye, the patient is taught to alternate. A 0.8 Bangerter foil is worn full time (20/30 VA level) for three to six months. Clear contact paper or scotch tape is worn three hours a day. The patient should schedule a return visit in six to eight weeks to check if improved vision in the amblyopic eye is maintained.

IMPORTANT: Some studies show two hours of patching is as effective as six hours. Furthermore, six hours of daily patching is as effective as full time (less one hour) daily patching. Other studies PEDIG (Pediatric Eye Disease Investigative Group) suggest six hours daily patching is similar to 12 hours daily patching. It also has been reported that two, four, and six hours and patching full time are similar. In addition, studies have shown that after cessation of treatment, 7% of children in this age group have recurrence of amblyopia.

IV. Amblyopia Treatment Ages Four to Twelve with Eccentric Fixation, Including Pleoptics

A. Treatment VA 20/200 or less

1. Initial Treatment

Full-time skin occlusion of the preferred eye during all waking hours. The patient is observed at three weeks intervals to evaluate:

a. the fixation pattern and visual acuity of the amblyopic eye, and,
b. the vision of the dominant eye being occluded.

In cases in which the child cannot accept occlusion of the good eye during school, the patch is transferred to the amblyopic eye and the dominant eye is patched after school and on weekends. The amblyopic eye must be occluded when the dominant eye is being used to prevent reinforcement of the eccentric area.

The occlusion program is continued as long as fixation or visual acuity improves. Once improvement remains stationary for two consecutive months, the second stage of treatment is based on the visual acuity and fixation achieved with full-time occlusion.

2. Treatment After Full-Time Occlusion of the Dominant Eye

a. 20/30 to 20/50 and good fixation

Fixation is central, central unsteady or minimal degree of eccentricity. Skin patch the preferred eye only half a day or full-time occlusion with 0.3 or 0.2 Bangerter Foil. The child should be observed in two to four weeks to monitor any change in visual acuity. If vision does diminish, return to full-time skin occlusion for an additional two months. (Correction of any significant refractive error should be worn full time). Make another attempt with ½ day skin occlusion for an additional two months to reinforce and stabilize the improved VA in the amblyopic eye. The management of the strabismic problem can now be initiated.

b. 20/60 to 20/80 vision with fixation is eccentric

The success of retaining 20/60 to 20/80 visual acuity is poor once occlusion is discontinued. However, the examiner can reassure the parents that if anything would happen to the dominant eye, the patient has reserved vision in the amblyopic eye (spare eye). The level of improvement can always be regained if needed during his or her life span.

c. 20/100 or less

If after three months of full-time occlusion, the vision has not improved to 20/100, stop the occlusion of the dominant eye and transfer patch to the amblyopic (eccentrically fixing) eye. The patch is worn full-time (waking hours) over the amblyopic eye for six to eight months to prevent stimulation or reinforcement of the eccentrically fixing area. Following this period of inverse patching, reinitiate full-time occlusion of the dominant eye for three additional months. If no improvement, stop treatment.

B. Treatment with Pleoptics for Eccentric Fixation

1. The amblyopic eye is constantly patched except when treatment is given.

2. Two methods of treatment with pleoptics are:

   a. Bangerter's Method-Instruments

      1. Pleoptophor with passive stimulation of the macula after dazzling the eccentric area. This instrument allows treatment for children in four to six age level.

      2. Corrector, Centrophore, Separator, Localizer and Memoscope are hand and eye memory practices to actively stimulate the macula.

   b. Cuppers' Method-Instruments

      1. Euthyscope (after-image technique): Re-educates the fovea to localize straight ahead.

      2. Koordinator, Space Koordinator, Ocular Synoptophore and Koordinator: contains the Haidinger Brushes which can only stimulate macula-papillar fibers of the macular area.

C. Binder's Red Filter Technique

The sound eye is occluded and a Wratten 92 red filter is taped to the plano or corrective spectacle lens in front of the eccentric eye and a shield is placed around the sides of the frame to prevent outside light from entering the amblyopic eye. Because of the familiar Purkinje phenomenon, the red light transmitted by the filter is much more heavily weighted for the excitation of cones in proportion to rods than is the case for the unfiltered visible light.

V. Pharmaceutical Penalization

An alternate method to patching in children with moderate amblyopia (20/50 to 20/80) studies has shown that in patients with central or unsteady central fixation, atropine penalization is as effective or better than patching. Children who patch initially improve more quickly than with atropine.

A. Method of Treatment

1. 1% atropine drops are instilled in the dominant eye

2. If a hyperopic correction is worn, remove lens in front of the dominant eye and replace with a plano lens.

3. Child is seen at three-week intervals as long as VA continues to improve. Stop atropine once improvement of VA remains the same for 2 consecutive months.

PEDIG studies show that using atropine two days during the week (weekend atropine) is as effective as using atropine daily in children with moderate amblyopia. Weekend use of atropine is also effective in children with severe amblyopia but the improvement is greater in younger children.

Vi. Additional Modalities of Treatment

If the optimum VA is not obtained with 1% atropine other modalities of treatment may be considered.

A. Bangerter foils - worn full-time in front of the dominant eye.

B. Optical penalization – increase *plus* lens in front of preferred eye.

C. Occlusion contact lens – over the dominant eye.

D. Clear contact paper or magic scotch tape in front of the dominant eye.

E. Levodopa/Carbidopa - oral medication with patching of the dominant eye.

F. Botulinum toxins – inducing ptosis in the sound eye.

G. Suturing a plastic occlusion shield over the sound eye.

Chapter 5

ESODEVIATION

An Esodeviation Is An Inward Turning Of One Eye

I. Latent Esodeviations - Comitant/Incomitant

A. General Information

Esophoria-latent inward deviation held in check by fusion. It may be comitant or incomitant. The amount of esophoria regarded as normal limits in adults is *2-3 prism diopters for distance* and near; normal range for children is slightly higher. *During illness, fatigue or emotional stress*, an esophoria may be intermittent.

Symptoms	Objectively –	watery appearance of eyes, congested conjunctiva.
	Subjectively –	headache, tiredness, rapid fatigue, blurriness of vision, symptoms associated with near work.

B. Types of Esophoria - Comitant

1. *Basic esophoria, intermittent esotropia* - recheck the refractive error.

   a. Characteristics
      1. Deviation equal in all gazes.
      2. NPC is normal.
      3. Convergence amplitudes are normal to high.
      4. Divergence amplitudes are low.
      5. Some suppression *usually present* (ET state).
      6. Good steropsis (but affected in ET state).

   b. Tests – cover test 6 m and 1/3 m, right – left, up and down gaze.

   c. Treatment – Only treat patients that have *symptoms.*

      1. Check the refractive error.
      2. Eliminate suppression, if present.

Teach diplopia in following situations, if *E(T)* is produced by testing procedure and suppression is demonstrated:

i. taking an NPC.
ii. doing red glass test distance and near.
iii. Worth Four Dot distance and near.
At the point where suppression is present, teach the patient to alternate with diplopia awareness with red glass and light. Place red filter in front of dominant eye at the point where suppression is present; flash your hand up and down in front of red filter eye until diplopia is elicited. If unable to maintain diplopia for fifty counts in the office, it is given as home practice five to ten minutes each day and a return visit in two or three weeks.

3. Stabilize fusion.

Once stable diplopia is elicited, the patient is given a red glass fusion practice. Begin where patient sees one fused (pink) image and advance (to 1/3 m) and recess (6 m) from that position. This practice is done in five minute sessions three times a day. Patient is seen in two to three weeks.

4. Additional anti-suppression.

Additional anti-suppression practices for distance and near fixation.

a. Framing - (phenomenon of physiologic diplopia) is an excellent distance practice. Have patient fix at a distant object and place a pencil or finger in front of his eyes. He should be aware of two pencils or two fingers as they fuse the distant object.

b. Bar reading – (phenomenon of physiologic diplopia) is an excellent near practice. While reading at near, hold a pencil (or finger or bar) in front of the book and patient should see two bars (or two fingers or two pencils) while reading. If he loses part of the page, suppression is present.

5. Increase amplitudes of fusion.

   Loose prisms are given as a home practice to increase relative fusional divergence and if indicated relative fusional convergence. The amount of base-in prism practice given is dependent upon the patient's performance in the office. The prism can be easily taped on the glasses. For example, if he blurs with a 3^{Δ} base-in prism with 20/30 target at distance but for near can accomplish a 10^{Δ} base-in; give the patient a 5^{Δ} base-in prism recession practice while looking at TV for 20 minutes each day (can break it up into five to ten minute intervals). Patient begins close to the TV to obtain a clear single picture and slowly moves away maintaining the image clear and single to six meters.

   IMPORTANT: If the patient has intermittent suppression while doing base-in prism practices, use physiologic diplopia awareness as a check mark for the patient. (He holds a finger or pencil in front of his eyes and observes two fingers or two pencils while fixing the object of regard; then if one finger or pencil disappears, suppression is present).

6. Fresnel press-on prisms management.

   If symptoms persist after normal amplitudes have been accomplished, the patient is given base-out Fresnel press-on prisms for the amount of esodeviation present. This method is used mainly in older children and adults. They are worn for two to three weeks as a trial period to evaluate improvement of symptoms. Should symptoms be relieved, slowly reduce strength of prism at $3\text{-}5^{\Delta}$ increments. If unsuccessful in reducing prism, permanent base-out prism in spectacles can be prescribed but the patient should be informed that the amount of base-out prism needed for comfortable binocular vision increases with passage of time.

7. Surgical management is dependent upon the amount of misalignment with or without press-on prism management

   Surgery: Check if eso greater looking at distance and near, right-left and up & down gaze at distance fixation.

2. Divergence Insufficiency Type (Eso greater at distance) – esophoria or intermittent esotropia.

   a. Etiology
   Primary disorder may be associated with *hypokinetic innervational* influences or *intrinsic* defects in ocular motor mechanism. It could easily be secondary to prolonged convergence excess or associated with under corrected hyperopia. Patients frequently demonstrate a nervous or psychic instability.

   b. Characteristics
      1. Usually of functional origin.
      2. Esodeviation greater for distance than near – increases with distance fixation.
      3. Comitant in all directions of gaze.
      4. Periods of fatigue may demonstrate ET with uncrossed diplopia.
      5. NPC normal.
      6. Minimal suppression.
      7. Prism divergence greatly reduced or absent.
      8. Prism convergence good.

   c. Treatment
      1. Check the refractive error.
      2. Give red glass and penlight recession practice 15 minutes daily.
      3. Another method is physiologic awareness beginning at near with TV and recess to 6 meters maintaining 2 fingers or pencils and a single image.
      4. Attempt to improve fusional divergence (BI recession practice) though frequently ineffective.

5. Give Fresnel press-on prism equal to the amount of esodeviation to evaluate improvement of symptoms. An attempt can be made to gradually reduce prism.

   NOTE: Since patient is ortho to minimal esophoria for near, the Fresnel prism is only placed on the upper segment of lens for distance fixation.

6. Surgical correction or ground-in prism may be considered.

3. Convergence Excess Type (esophoria – intermittent esotropia) – greater for near.

   a. Characteristics
      1. Associated with excessive accommodation or an abnormally high convergence response to accommodative impulse – high AC/A.
      2. Esophoria greater for near than for distance.
      3. NPC normal.
      4. Convergence amplitude normal.
      5. Divergence amplitude usually low, especially at near.
      6. Suppression is frequently present.

   b. Measurements

      Measure the alignment with +1.00, +2.00, +3.00 add OU for near with accommodative target and repeat primary position measurement to evaluate the minimal strength needed to obtain stable fusion at distance and near.

   c. Treatment

      Same as for basic esophoria with these modifications:

      1. Physiologic diplopia. Since the angle of deviation is greater at near and the fusional ability of the patient is greatly taxed, the introduction of any obstacle to binocularity (the object on which he is to appreciate physiologic diplopia) may cause a manifest deviation. Have the patient relax while looking at a distance object and gradually introduce a small stick (pick-up stick or Q-tip) in the midline close to the nose.

Gradually move the stick away from the patient to that distance where he is able to appreciate it in physiologic diplopia. If he crosses inward, move the stick back to the area of his nose and repeat until control is mastered. If the patient's fusional control is too unstable to perform this exercise, additional plus lenses for near should be given in an effort to control the deviation and allow fusion of a sufficiently stable quality to permit binocular training.

2. Increase fusional amplitude with emphasis on relative fusion divergence with base-in prism or minus lenses.

3. Bifocals may be prescribed by the ophthalmologist for those patients with a high latent deviation at near which, after maximum improvement of divergence amplitudes, continue to have symptoms or easily break down into an intermittent esotropia.

4. Plus lenses may be reduced gradually as quality of binocularity and fusional divergence amplitudes improve. Reduction of plus lenses is given *only* if the patient demonstrates no sacrifice of binocular function or discomfort with the weaker lenses.

5. Prisms are not generally prescribed for this condition except for press-on prism test preoperatively.

II. Manifest Esodeviations – Comitant Types

A. Congenital or Infantile Esotropia - Tonic-Type, constantly present under ordinary circumstances, but completely relieved by anesthesia.

1. Characteristic
    a. Early onset – within first three months of life.
    b. Variable angle of squint but usually not accommodative.
    c. May have moderate hyperopia.
    d. Large deviation – 40^{Δ} or greater prism diopters of esotropia – may have vertical deviation as well.
    e. Frequently alternating. If uniocular, amblyopia is usually present.
    f. Cross fixation.

g. No evidence of paresis.
h. ARC and suppression may be present.

2. Treatment
   a. Refraction – 1% Cyclogyl.
   b. Patch to overcome amblyopia (*check fixation and following pattern*) and induced tropia test.
   c. Skin patch 4-6 hours a day – check at weekly intervals under *one year* of age and at two week intervals at two years or older. Continue patch program until good fixation with either eye before surgical management.
   d. Early surgery (3-4 months of age) is recommended. The procedure can be bimedial recessions or a recession-resection of one eye.
   e. If further surgery is indicated, usually within 3 months of last surgery.

B. Congenital or Infantile Esotropia – associated with high degree of myopia.

1. Etiology

Innervational type of strabismus associated with uncorrected high myopia. Convergent position of eyes allows good vision at near and child remains in eso position at all distances.

a. Characteristics
   1. Moderate to high myopia.
   2. Deep suppression, especially at distance fixation.

b. Treatment
   1. Give full minus correction. Refract again in three months to uncover more myopia if present.
   2. Wear correction at least six months. In most instances, child becomes straight with good fusion.

C. Orthoptics

1. Amblyopia – patch preferred eye three to four hours a day; check at weekly intervals until fixation is central and child can voluntarily fix with previous amblyopic eye.

2. Alternate the skin patch two to three hours a day to teach alternation.

3. Once good alternation is achieved, surgical management depends upon the amount of residual deviation. If the deviation is 15^{Δ} or greater press-on prism may be considered for one to two weeks to determine fusion potential.

4. If fusion or no fusion – surgical management depends upon the total amount of esodeviation with or without press-on prism management.

D. Accommodative Esotropia

Etiology is the relationship of accommodation to convergence. Whenever accommodation occurs, there is a *related amount* of convergence and the manner in which convergence is expressed is dependent on several factors.

E. Accommodative Esotropia – with normal AC/A ratio

This informs us that the child has an uncorrected hyperopia and he has to accommodate more than the normal (emmetropic) person for clear distance vision. *Accommodation* brings forth *accommodative convergence* in *proportion* to the patient's *AC/A ratio* and the amount of his *hypermetropia. Accommodative convergence* brought forth by accommodation would be in excess of that required for *bifoveal fixation.* If his amplitude of *relative fusional* divergence is insufficient to overcome this excessive convergence, esotropia will result each time *accommodation is exerted.* Since the AC/A ratio is normal, the situation for near is approximately the same as for distance. The angle of deviation will vary with the amount of accommodation exerted.

1. Characteristics

   a. Due to uncorrected hyperopia 2D to 5D.
   b. Relatively late onset – age two to three years.
   c. Intermittent at first – evident when child is tired, ill or upset.
   d. Deviation about the same for distance and near.
   e. Moderate angle esotropia (25-35 prism diopters).

f. Because the angle is unstable and intermittent, ARC is not present.
g. Suppression usually present - with anisometropia.
h. Rarely amblyopia – except in children with anisometropia.
i. NPC to nose.
j. Fusion is demonstrated on the Synoptophore.
k. Convergence amplitudes good to excessive.
l. Divergence amplitudes fair to poor.

2. Testing - Initial orthoptic visit

   a. Cover test: use 20/30 target at 6 m and measure in primary position in addition to up, down, right and left gaze. At near on accommodative target at near with and without +3.00 clip-on's.
   b. Red glass test for distance and near and Worth Four Dot flashlight at distance and near (check stereo with and without +3.00 add).
   c. Amblyoscope findings if available.

3. Treatment

   a. Cyclogyl 1% refraction up to teenage age.
   b. Give full hyperopic correction under school age and minimum hyperopic correction that allows *comfortable binocular vision* in school age children.

      i. If amblyopia is present, hyperoptic correction is worn full-time for four to six weeks before initiating amblyopia treatment. In the majority of cases, once the eyes are aligned with the proper hyperoptic correction, visual acuity improves in the previously amblyopic eye.

      ii. Eliminate amblyopia (usually minimal) by initiating skin occlusion or placing clear contact paper on the lens in front of the preferred eye. This is worn three to four hours daily until VA is equal to the good eye. Bangerter foils, which are worn full-time, could be considered as an alternate method in amblyopia patient.

iii. Anti-suppression practice with the red filter and penlight is excellent if only intermittent diplopia is present. This can be performed 20 minutes daily at five minute intervals with the red filter in front of the preferred eye and maintain a single pink (red and white mixed) from to the bridge of the nose to a distance of six meters. Have the child do additional exercises such as red drawing, coloring, beading, etc., with the red filter over the preferred eye.

iv. Physiologic diplopia awareness can be while looking at TV from 1/3 meter to six meters if suppression continues to be a problem.

v. Patient is seen at three to four week intervals until VA is equal and comfortable and stable fusion is maintained with good stereopsis. Patient can be monitored at three to four month intervals and refraction should be performed yearly.

vi. On return visit for a yearly refraction, determine if the *plus* lens can be reduced. Begin with 1.00 clip-on lens and wait at least 20 minutes to determine if equal VA is maintained with stable fusion at distance and near.

vii. Residual esotropia is still present with the first prescription, check if more plus is indicated (+1.00 clips). If no change and the angle of esotropia is less than 12 prism diopter, equal VA, with or without peripheral fusion, just monitor the patient at four to six month intervals. If the residual ET is 20^{Δ} or greater, with or without fusion potential, additional surgery may be considered.

F. Accommodative Esotropia – with high AC/A ratio (convergence-excess)

1. Etiology

   The refractive error in this type of esotropia is not the primary factor. These patients may be *emmetropic, hyperopic,* or even *myopic.* It is common, however, to see a *moderate hypermetropic refractive error.*

   Characterized by a high AC/A ratio, the excessive convergence for near may be due to a general weakness of accommodation (hypoaccommodation) or it may be due to excessive accommodation to convergence responses.

   IMPORTANT: Observe in causal seeing – patient may be phoric or intermittent.

2. Characteristics
   a. Relatively late onset – age two to three years.
   b. Deviation is greater for near *(10-15) prism diopters).*
   c. Remote *NPA* but not always present.
   d. Amblyopia is rare due to *variability of the angle.*
   e. Convergence amplitude high to normal.
   f. Divergence amplitudes low.
   g. Suppression more common than with normal AC/A ratio-type deviation. (Suppression in ET state especially for near.)

3. Treatment
   a. Proper correction of refractive error.
   b. Bifocals in amount necessary to provide *bifoveal fusion* for near. (+2.50 or +3.00 executive type at lower pupillary margin).
   c. Anti-suppression practices.
      i. Doing red work, drawing, coloring, etc. with red filter over preferred eye looking through bifocal.
      ii. Do physiological diplopia awareness while reading through the bifocal holding pencil in front of the page.
   d. Increase relative fusional *divergence with base-in prism* through bifocal. If concerned that patient may suppress with prism practice, have him be aware of physiologic diplopia while reading through bifocals.

e. Reduction of bifocals – reduction of bifocals usually begins at ages six to seven years. This could easily be performed in the office. Place a -1.00 sphere clip on lens OU in the office and have patient wear them 20 minutes in the waiting room, if phoric thru the bifocal, a permanent reduction in bifocal lens is prescribed.

   If still ET with -1.00 sphere clip then attempt to reduce bifocal in another six months. In cases in which bifocals cannot be eliminated, surgery may be considered in early teens.

G. Acquired Esotropia

Could have had a period of *bifoveal single vision* before deviation became manifested. Accommodative, motor, or innervational anomalies could have caused the esotropia but frequently an optical deficiency is usually the case in this group (eg. anisometropia, uncorrected accommodative ET).

1. Characteristics
   a. Age of onset one to five years.
   b. May be hyperopic but esotropia not relieved with glasses.
   c. Frequently *alternates* but when uniocular, suppression and amblyopia are often present.
   d. ARC may be present especially in a constant angle.
   e. Angle of deviation steadily increases because of secondary contraction of the muscle and is usually large (35^{Δ} or greater).
   f. No paresis present and is relieved by anesthesia.

2. Treatment (Check the refractive error.)
   a. Overcome amblyopia (occlusion as discussed in amblyopia lecture).
   b. Surgery is determined:
      i. Amount of deviation D&N, right, left, up and down gaze at distance.
      ii. Presence or absence of fusion – evaluate with the synoptophore or press-on prisms to prognosticate sensory or motor response.
      iii. If ARC – more aggressive surgical procedures

3. Postop Treatment
   a. 15^{Δ} or less phoric to intermittent esodeviation. Just follow at two to three month intervals. If concerned with suppression, teach patient physiologic diplopia awareness and increase relative fusional divergence and convergence amplitudes with BI and BO prisms.
   b. 20^{Δ} or greater. Initiate base-out press-on prisms to prognosticate the presence of fusion and potential for good alignment. Patient is seen in one or two weeks to evaluate the response to decide surgical management.

   IMPORTANT: In postop secondary XT – reduce the plus correction. If reduction in plus is unsuccessful, press-on prisms can be considered to determine surgery management.

H. Nonaccommodative Esotropia

Due to anatomical anomalies or to an early paresis which has become comitant.

1. Characteristics
   a. Early onset.
   b. Deviation generally large (40^{Δ} or more) and usually basic type.
   c. May be uniocular or alternating.
   d. Deep suppression and amblyopia may be present.
   e. ARC may be present because of a constant angle.

2. Management
   a. Check refractive error.
   b. Treat amblyopia and suppression as previously described in amblyopia section in children.
   c. In adult patients consider press-on prisms to determine the sensory and motor response preoperatively.
   d. *Surgery is determined for total amount of esodeviation.*

3. Post-op Treatment - Similar to acquired esotropia group.

I. Mixed-type Esotropia.
Referred to as partially accommodative Esotropia.

1. Characteristics

Comprised of an accommodative and nonaccommodative components. Same characteristics as in accommodative Esotropia and nonaccommodative Esotropia except the residual deviation (nonaccommodative portion) may vary from a small to moderate nonaccommodative angle of esodeviation.

2. Treatment
As indicated for component parts, as outlined in Accommodative and Nonaccommodative Esotropia.

a. Wear full hyperopic correction for two months.
b. Eliminate amblyopia – follow amblyopia lecture.
c. Surgery is performed for the nonaccommodative portion (residual ET with hyperopia correction). Press-on prisms may be useful to determine fusion potential preoperatively.
d. Post-op treatment – follow same post-op treatment for acquired ET.

J. Phoria-Tropia or Monofixation Esotropia

Sometimes called: Monofixation syndrome, micro-strabismus, phoria-tropia, ET flick, retinal slip.

1. Characteristics
a. Less than 10 prism diopters of heterotropia. With simultaneous prism and cover test, usually $2\text{-}6^{\Delta}$.
b. Angle increases with alternate cover test.
c. VA is often one line lower in the non-fixing eye.
d. Stereopsis is present (usually not more than 67%).
e. May be central or slightly eccentric on visuscope or ophthalmoscope.
f. Harmonious ARC.
g. Demonstrates a three degree facultative scotoma in visual field of non-fixing eye during binocular fixation.
h. Fusional vergences are present.

2. Causes
   a. Strabismic history.
   b. Anisometropia.
   c. Uniocular macular lesion.
   d. Amblyopia.
   e. Eccentric fixation.

3. Tests
   a. Simultaneous prism and cover with prism over non-fixing eye.
   b. 4 Base-out Test – absence of movement is interpreted as proof of scotoma (out movement not in).
   c. Worth 4 Dot – claims four for near, demonstrate suppression for distance.

4. Treatment

   If no symptoms, leave alone. If symptoms, increase fusional amplitudes from subjective angle on synoptophore. Also can be done in free spaces with BI and BO prisms with the small tropia – just look at re-fixation movement.

K. Blind Spot Syndrome

Condition may occur spontaneously or following a surgically reduced large angle esotropia or over-corrected XT. An accommodative element may or may not be present. There are *no* associated sensory anomalies.

1. Characteristics
   a. ET 12 to 18 degrees (25-35 prism diopters), may have coexistent vertical deviation up to 10 prism diopters.
   b. Good vision in each eye.
   c. NRC.
   d. Fusion demonstrated on the synoptophore; frequently with stereopsis and amplitudes.
   e. No suppression, diplopia easily recognized when prism is placed before the deviating eye and the image is displaced out of the blind spot.
   f. Transitory diplopia may be present.
   g. Easily confirmed with Lancaster Red-Green Test which is a fovea-to-fovea test.

3. Treatment
   a. Correct hyperopia if present.
   b. Place a base-out press-on prism in front of the preferred eye or equally in front of both eyes in the amount to neutralize or slightly over-correct the deviation. In this way, the patient is fusing constantly pre-op and establishing amplitudes of fusion.
   c. Orthoptic office treatment can be given on the synoptophore (from the objective angle) to increase relative fusional divergence and convergence amplitudes.
   d. Surgery.

L. Blind Spot Mechanism

Mechanism differs from the syndrome by presence of sensory anomalies.

1. Characteristics
   a. ET 12 to 18 degrees (25-35$^{\Delta}$) with possible vertical deviation up to 5 prism diopters.
   b. Suppression, amblyopia, ARC or a combination of the three present.

2. Treatment
   a. Correct refractive error.
   b. Treat amblyopia.
   c. Teach alternation.
   d. To evaluate preop alignment, place BO press-on prism in front of preferred eye in children and non-preferred eye in adults in amount to neutralize or slightly over-correct deviation. Surgery is determined on the total amount of prisms prescribed.

M. Lancaster Red-Green Test

Diagnostic Method of Confirming the Blind Spot Syndrome or Mechanism

1. To determine if image of the deviated eye falls in the blind spot with the Lancaster Red-Green Test:

a. Place the patient at a distance of 1 meter from the tangent screen. Determine the blind spot in the visual field for each eye and plot it on the screen. This is a fovea to fovea test.
b. Patient is give red-green goggles (red-OD, green-OS) and one of the hand torches (e.g. red) is held by the patient and the other (e.g. green) torch is held by the examiner. The light held by the examiner (e.g. green) determines the fixing eye.
c. The examiner places his green light straight ahead at 0 and the patient is asked to superimpose his red light on the green light.
d. If the patient place his red light in the blind spot (plotted on the tangent screen) of the left eye, a blind spot syndrome or mechanism is present.

III. Manifest Esodeviations – Incomitant Types

A. Strabismus Fixus

1. Etiology
Due to *rigid, fibrous, short medial rectus muscle* attached by a *broad fibrous area to the sclera near the equator.* Fixes the eye in a position of adduction with *complete loss of abduction.*

2. Characteristics
a. It is *congenital.*
b. Both eyes in *adducted position*_(one may be *affected more than the other*) with *50+$^{\Delta}$ ET.*
c. Absence or extreme limitation of *abduction.*
d. *Restricted rotations externally on forced duction.*
e. Cross-fixation present.
f. *May be limitation of elevation and depression.*
g. *Compensates for lack of lateral rotation* with head movements.

3. Treatment - Surgery

B. Nystagmus Blockage Syndrome

Rare cause early onset of comitant esotropia

1. Onset of esotropia in early infancy-described by Cuppers.
2. Pseudo-abducens paralysis.
3. Head turn toward the side of the fixating eye.
4. Absence of nystagmus with the fixating eye in adduction.
5. Appearance of a manifest nystagmus as the fixating eye moved into primary position and abduction.
6. Convergence blocks the nystagmus.
7. Esotropia is caused by sustained convergence and secondary changes in the medial rectus muscle.

C. Ciancia Syndrome

1. Described in 1962 as a syndrome of infantile esotropia with abduction nystagmus.
2. ET early onset.
3. Large angle ET.
4. Bilateral limitation of abduction.
5. Jerk nystagmus with quick phase toward the side of fixating eye.
6. Increase in abduction and disappearing in adduction.
7. Torticollis with face turn toward side of fixating eye.
8. Moderate or absent hyperopia.
9. Head tilting toward side of fixating eye.

Summary: Ciancia syndrome, nystagmus blockage and large angle congenital esotropia – very sensitive characteristics and may be part of the spectrum of same condition.

D. Paretic Esotropia (Recent Onset - Abducens Palsy/6th Nerve Palsy/Lateral Rectus Palsy)

1. Characteristics
   a. Angle of squint varies with each eye fixing and varies in fields of gaze.
   b. Limitation of the lateral rectus muscle or overshoot of medial rectus on horizontal gaze.
   c. Compensatory head posture to eliminate diplopia.
   d. Past-pointing present due to diplopia.
   e. NRC is present.
   f. Symptoms are diplopia, vertigo, dizziness, nausea, etc. These symptoms rapidly disappear in children but last in varying degrees in adults. It rarely is permanent except with a neuropathic type of patient.

2. Treatment
   a. Use press-on prism in front of the paretic eye to prevent secondary contracture in the amount to neutralize the deviation. If patient is too young or too uncomfortable with prisms, alternate patch to eliminate diplopia.
   b. Wait until deviation stabilizes. Usually six months but it may be as long as one year.
   c. Surgery.

E. Paretic Esotropia (long-standing)

1. Characteristics
   a. Measurements become comitant with time.
   b. Secondary contracture may be present but rare in congenital cases.
   c. No past-pointing present since no diplopia present.
   d. Suppression, amblyopia (deepness depends on age of onset) and ARC may be present.
   e. Compensatory head posture may not be present.

2. Treatment
   a. Eliminate suppression and amblyopia as indicated in previous lectures in children.
   b. If ARC present, must be more aggressive in surgical management.

c. If fusion potential is questionable, attempt a two to four week trial with press-on prisms as described in *Acquired Esotropia.*
d. Surgery.

3. Postop Treatment
b. If fusion is present, stabilize with BI and BO prism amplitude training.
c. No fusion: If VA is equal and angle of deviation is 20^{Δ} or less with SPCT the patient looks acceptable cosmetically, further treatment not indicated. The patient may establish gross fusion at this smaller angle.
d. If cosmetically not acceptable, an additional procedure is done on the opposite eye.

F. Duane's Retraction Syndrome

1. Etiology

In typical patients, it is generally though that the lateral rectus of the affected eye is replaced by a fibrotic band. In some instances, fibrous medial recti have been found. Investigation has shown electromyography has led to the conclusion that in most cases there is a super nuclear lesion (simultaneous stimulation of both the lateral rectus and medial rectus muscles cranial 3rd nerve afferently innervates lateral rectus) present alone or in combination with abnormality of the muscle.

2. Characteristics
a. Patient may or may not have a minimal to a significant face turn to the side of the affected eye.
b. Good fusion usually present.
c. Abduction of the affected eye is nil or limited to a few degrees past midline.
e. Minimal restriction of adduction of the affected eye on versions and forced ductions.
f. Retraction of globe on attempted adduction.
g. Narrowing of palpebral fissure on adduction of affected eye; widening on attempted abduction.
h. Upshoot or downshoot of the affected eye on adduction.
i. Usually unilateral, may be bilateral.
i. In some case, may have reversed findings, Type II.

3. Treatment

Surgery, if patient has a significant face turn.

Type I -	Widening of palpebral fissure on attempted abduction. Narrowing of palpebral fissure on attempted adduction with retraction of the globe. Esophoria, Intermittent ET, Esotropia
Type II –	Widening of palpebral fissure on attempted abduction and narrowing on attempted adduction with retraction of the globe - XT. Exophoria, Intermittent XT and Exotropia.
Type III –	No abduction or adduction and narrowing and widening of palpebral fissure still present. Minimal to no deviation in primary position - ET or XT.

Chapter 6

ACCOMMODATION AND CONVERGENCE

AC/A RATIO

I. Accommodation

The process by which the dioptic power of the eye may be altered by changes of convexity of the crystalline lens. Process is accomplished by contraction of the ciliary muscle allows the fibers of the zonules to relax and the lens in the elastic capsule becomes thicker and more relaxed, thus accommodation occurs. The unit used to express the refraction of the eye is the *diopter* (D). It designates the refractive power of the lens which is equal to the reciprocal of the lens focal length in meters. Two *diopter* lenses bring parallel rays of light to focus at ½ m.

The amount of change in the refractive power of the eye brought about by accommodation gradually decreases with age, ranging from about 20 D. in the very young child to 1 D. at approximately age 60. This process called presbyopia usually becomes clinically significant about the age of 40-45 at which time bifocals for near work are usually required.

With respect to the emmetropic eye, light rays emanating from an object point within infinity (20 ft. or 6m. for practical purposes) are divergent on striking the retina thus producing a blurred image. To bring these divergent rays to a point focus coincident with the retina, the dioptric power of the eye must be increased sufficiently by accommodation unless lenses are used. The exact nature of the stimulus by means of which the blurred image on the retina gives rise to the accommodation reflex is not entirely known but the resultant accommodation occurs with great precision and is generally completed in about half a second.

II. Clinical Measurements of Accommodation

A. *Far point* of accommodation-the axial point is conjugate with retina axial point in the un-accommodative eye. It is the most distant point from the eye an object is seen clearly. Example:

1. Far point of the emmetropic eye is at infinity.
2. Far point of the myopic eye is in front of the eye.
3. Far point of the hyperopic eye is a virtual point behind the eye.

B. *Near point* of accommodation (NPA) Nearest point of clear vision-position closest to the eye where a small print can be kept in sharp focus by maximum accommodation.

C. *Amplitude of accommodation* - difference express in diopters (D) between *far* point and *near* point of accommodation.

D. *Measurement* of amplitudes of accommodation. A = F-N

A = is the amplitude of accommodation.

F = the vergence of light rays corresponding to the far point – is the most distant point from the eye an object is seen clearly.

N = the vergence of near point rays at the eye-nearest point letter can be seen.

Clinically is performed separately with each eye.

1. Full correction worn – place Prince rule – outside temporal corner of the eye
2. Small print close to the eye – and moved back until clear – *far point*
3. Nearest point letter can be seen – *near point* (use Prince rule). Binocular reading usually indicates a nearer *NPA*.
4. The size test type to be used should correlate with the patient's corrected visual acuity for distance. If the Prince rule or similar device is used for this test, the near point of accommodation in centimeters, the amplitude of accommodation in diopters, and the normal amplitude of accommodation by age are readily determined. All three scales are marked on the rule.

III. Convergence

A. *Voluntary convergence* – volitional rotation of the eyes, nasalwards.

This is the only dysjunctive movement of the eyes which can be initiated at will. The exact location of the cortical center for voluntary convergence is not known.

B. *Involuntary convergence* – psycho-optical reflex on fixation and refixation reflexes.

Requires cooperation of the cortex in the act of attention.

Involuntary convergence is divided in four types:

1. *Tonic* – Brings eyes from the usual divergence of rest to parallelism in primary position – Static
2. *Accommodative* – convergence reflex brought forth in response to accommodation to obtain a clear single image
3. *Fusional* convergence brought about in interest of fusion to overcome diplopia – Dynamic
4. *Proximal* – convergence resulting from awareness of a near object – Dynamic, eg. (Synoptophore) – machine convergence

C. *Near* point of convergence – nearest point object is seen clearly.

1. objectively – penlight to nose
2. subjectively – patient sees double
3. red glass and light test

D. *Amplitude* of convergence – Maximum amount of convergence which can be obtained while binocularity is present.

Absolute fusional convergence- amount of convergence which can be exerted irrespective of state of accommodation.

Relative fusional convergence – Amount of convergence which can be exerted while accommodation remains constant.

E. Units used in measurement of convergence.

1. Prism diopter – Δ 1 prism diopter will displace a ray of light 1 cm at 1 meter distant

2. Meter angle (M.A.) – angular use of convergence

   One meter angle is the amount of convergence required to binocularity fixation at 1 m away equal to the reciprocal of distance (in meters) between the object and bridge of the nose. Value varies directly with interpupillary distance.

   Conversion of M.A. to Δ's – multiply the number of M.A.'s by the interpupillary distance expressed in cm, eg,

   1 M.A. = 6^{Δ} with 6 cm PD at 1 M
   1/3 M = $6^{\Delta} \times 3 = 18^{\Delta}$ at 1/3 M

F. *Near* Reflex

When looking at a close object, an innervation to contract is sent simultaneously to ciliary muscle for accommodation, to M R muscle for convergence and sphincter papillae for pupillary constriction to obtain a clear image.

IV. AC/A Ratio – Accommodation Relationship

Convergence Relationship is a very tight, linear one

A. For each *impulse* for a change in *accommodation* there is a corresponding impulse for change in convergence.

B. For each individual an *impulse* for a certain amount of *accommodation* reflex brings forth a *precise quantity* of *accommodative convergence* in a *consistent ratio,* which is *peculiar and stable* in the individual relationship - this is termed the AC/A ratio.

AC = accommodation convergence in prism diopters or meter angle
A = accommodation in diopters

AC/A ratio is accommodative convergence in prism diopters associated per diopter of accommodation.

C. Normal AC/A Ratio

Ideally, the quantity of accommodation convergence reflexively associated with that amount of accommodation required for clear vision at any fixation distance would allow exact bifoveal fixation.

However, seldom does this occur. Usually, there is a slight deficit and occasionally an overabundance of accommodative convergence, which must be either augmented or overcome by employing fusional vergences. In cases of a normal AC/A ratio, the fusional amplitudes can usually successfully offset this discrepancy.

The normal AC/A ratio expressed in meter angles of convergence is 1 M.A./1D, i.e., for a fixation distance of 1/3 M. the 3 D of accommodation required for clear vision is reflexively associated with 3 M.A. of convergence, giving a ratio of 1 M.A./1D.

From a clinical standpoint, the deviation of patients with a normal AC/A is found to be nearly equal for distance and near. Normal AC/A ratio is 4-5^{Δ}/1D.

D. Abnormally High AC/A Ratio

In some cases, the amount of accommodative convergence brought forth in response to accommodation is excessively high. These are designated as having high AC/A ratios. Two theories have been postulated regarding these cases:

1. The convergence mechanism is highly responsive to accommodative stimuli.

2. There is a weakness of the accommodation mechanism, which requires excessive innervation to bring about the desired accommodation and this affects an excessive accommodative response. AC/A ratios as high as 10^{Δ} to 12^{Δ} have been recorded.

   Clinically, the deviation of patients with an abnormally high AC/A ratio is found to be more esotropic (or less exotropic) as near than at distance; the near deviation approximates the distance deviation when measured with +3.00 D lens OU.

V. Measurement of AC/A Ratio

(Absolute Value)

1. Gradient method – $AC/A = \left(\frac{|\Delta_1 - \Delta|}{D} \right)$ (Absolute Value)

   Δ = original deviation
   Δ_1 = deviation measurement with lens
   D = power of lenses

   Example:
   Δ (original deviation) = esophoria 17

   Δ_1 (deviation with +3 lens) = esophoria 2

   D lens of 3D $\quad AC/A = \left(\frac{|2-(+17)|}{3} \right) = 5^{\Delta}/1D$

2. Heterophoria method

   $$AC/A = PD + \left(\frac{\Delta N - \Delta o}{D} \right)$$

   PD = pupillary distance (cm)
   ΔN = deviation for near
   Δo = deviation for 6 m
   D = fixation distance

   Example:

   PD = 6 cm
   ΔN = esophoria 17
   Δo = esophoria 2
   D = 33.3 cm (3D)

$$AC/A = 6 + \left(\frac{(+17)-(+2)}{3} \right) = 6 + \left(\frac{(17-2)}{3} \right) = 11\ D$$

Note: If no difference in D&N measurements – AC/A is the same as PD in cm.

Note: Abnormal high AC/A ratio accommodative convergence brought forth in response to accommodation is excessively high.

Two theories for high AC/A ratio:

(1) Convergence mechanism is highly responsive to accommodation stimuli.
(2) Weakness in accommodation mechanism requires excessive innervation to bring about the desired accommodation.

VI. Examples

Normal and High AC/A Ratio

ET sc = 16	Rx + 3.00	E = cc = 1
ET' sc = 16		E'= cc = 1

AC/A ratio (gradient)
AC/A ratio (heterophoria) = (PD 50 cm)

Accommodative ET With High AC/A Ratio

	E sc = 2	AC/A ratio (gradient)
	ET' sc = 23	AC/A ratio (heterophoria) – PD 50 cm
+2.00	E cc = 2	

VII. Clinical Method in Determining AC/A Ratio

A. Clinical method:

1. If a refractive error is present, it should be fully corrected.
2. Have patient fix a 20/30 target at six meters.
3. Measure the full amount of deviation with the prism and alternate cover tests.
4. Re-measure the deviation with a -1.00 diopter sphere placed in front of both eyes over the correction.
5. The difference in the amount of deviation between the first and second measurement represents the AC/A ratio.

Chapter 7

EXODEVIATION

I. Introduction

A. Etiology

The same for Exophoria, Intermittent Exotropia, and Exotropia.

1. Anatomical
   Divergent position of the orbits, divergent position of the rest or abnormal insertions of muscle and check ligaments.

2. Optical
   Defective vision in one eye occurring after childhood or in very early infancy.

3. Accommodative
   Secondary to weak or infrequently used accommodation
   a. Accommodation not used with presbyopic correction.
   b. Uncorrected astigmatism or uncorrected myopia (no accommodation needed for clear near vision).
   c. Uncorrected high or moderate hyperopia with fatigue from accommodative effort or problem with hypo-accommodation.
   d. Evidence of hypo-accommodation would be seen in patients with low accommodation, accommodation ratio, or low accommodation amplitudes. The Brückner test would reveal if a patient was not accommodating with a light crescent seen in the upper portion of the red reflex.

4. Neurogenic
   a. Paresis of an adductor.
   b. Disturbance of central innervations controlling convergence and divergence.

B. Measurements

Measurements for all exo patients in primary position should be done at *infinity*, 6 meters, 1/3 meter. Up, down, right and left gazes only at 6 meters.

II. Comitant Manifest Exodeviation

A. Exophoria and Intermittent Exotropia

1. Basic Exophoria and Intermittent Exotropia

The amount of deviation with fusion suspended and with eyes in the un-accommodated state. The amount of deviation is the same for both distances and near.

a. Characteristics
- ii. Onset relatively late, common especially in adults.
- iii. Asthenopia.
- iv. Exophoria is equal for distance and near.
- v. NPC remote or normal.
- vi. Convergence amplitudes low.
- vii. Divergence amplitudes normal but can be low.
- viii. Suppression present in varying degrees (tropic state).

b. Treatment
- i. Proper correction of refractive error – astigmatism and myopia fully corrected, check for hypoaccommodation in hyperopia and minimally correct presbyopia.

- ii. Teach diplopia at the distance the patient is tropic or in older children and adults teach physiological diplopia awareness while maintaining a fused image.

c. Method of Teaching Diplopia with Red Filter and Penlight.

- i. At the point when suppression occurs either at distance or near teach the patient diplopia awareness. Red filter is placed in front of dominant eye and patient fixates at a penlight, the examiner flashes his own hand in front of the unfiltered eye until diplopia is elicited. The patient is asked to hold the diplopia for 50 counts, if unsuccessful in office give this exercise for home training but diplopia should be held for 100 counts. This home practice is performed for a total of 10 minutes daily, five days a week. Patient is seen in two to three weeks.

ii. Stabilize fusion.
Once stable diplopia is elicited, then red glass fusion practice is given from the bridge of the nose to 6 meters away. Begin where patient sees one fused (pink) image and advance and recess from that position. This practice is done in five minute sessions three times a day. Patient returns in three weeks.

iii. Physiologic diplopia with anti-suppression practices for distance and near fixation.
   a. *Framing* - is an excellent distance practice. Have patient fix at a distant object and place a pencil or finger in front of his eyes. He or she should be aware of 2 pencils or 2 fingers as he fuses the distant object. If the patient is having difficulty seeing 2 fingers or pencils, shake finger or pencil briskly until he or she appreciates physiological diplopia. The patient starts at near to obtain a single picture on the TV and recesses back to 6 meters.
   b. *Bar reading* – is an excellent near practice. While reading at near, hold a pencil (or finger or bar) in front of the book and patient should see 2 bars (or 2 fingers or 2 pencils) while reading. If he loses part of the page, suppression is present. These practices are performed 15 minutes a day.

iv. Increase relative fusional convergence amplitudes.
Once stable fusion is achieved with the above eye exercises, initiate loose base-out prisms taped to the spectacles and if no correction buy sunglasses and remove lenses. Begin with a 5^{Δ} base-out prism and gradually increase the prism strength to 20 prism diopters. Begin at the distance single clear image is achieved and maintain fusion to a distance of 6 m to 1/3 m.

v. Fresnel press-on prisms management.
If symptoms persist after normal amplitudes have been accomplished, the patient is given base-in Fresnel press-on prisms for the amount of exodeviation present. This method is used mainly in older children

and adults. They are worn for 1-2 weeks as a trial period to evaluate improvement of symptoms. Should symptoms be relieved, slowly reduce strength of the prism. If unsuccessful in reducing the prism, permanent base-in prism in spectacles may be considered but are usually not recommended, since in most cases the amount of base-in prism needed for comfortable binocular vision increases with passage of time.

vi. Surgery management is usually considered for the total amount of exodeviation.

2. Intermittent Exotropia - Divergence Excess Type

Deviation greater at distance and may be a constant. This type of deviation is greater at distance, may be phoric or intermittent for near. If tropic at distance and phoric for near, it is called periodic exotropia.

a. Measurements
Measure the patient in primary position at *infinity*, 6 meters and 1/3 meter, up-down, right-left gazes.

In divergence excess type additional measurements with +3.00 at near (1/2 hour) to check if deviation increases due to accommodative convergence or occlusion at near (1/2 hour) to determine if measurements increase due to fusional mechanism. This differentiates between simulated divergence excess and an actual divergence excess type.

b. Characteristics
i. Gradual onset, usually early but may be later.
ii. Usually closes one eye in sunlight.
iii. X or XT greater at distance; less exodeviation or orthophoria for near. (Deviation at 200 feet greater than at 20 feet).
iv. Deviation at distance may be X (T) or XT.
v. NPC may be normal.
vi. Convergence amplitudes normal for near, distance convergence poor to good with or without suppression at break-point.
vii. Divergence amplitudes could be excessive to poor.

viii. Amblyopia is rare; suppression more frequent at distance.
ix. Possible overaction of the lateral rectus.

c. Treatment – Two methods of therapy

i. Alternate occlusion or occlusion of the preferred eye if amblyopia is present. This method prevents reinforcement of suppression and enhances stable fusion. Patient wears the patch four to six hours a day, followed at two month intervals. If stable fusion is not achieved in six months the patient is a candidate for surgical management.

ii. Increase relative fusional convergence with physiologic diplopia awareness if suppression is present.

A base-out prism is selected in the office. For example, if the patient can fuse a 5^{Δ} base-out prism at near but not at distance, the patient is sent home with a loose 5^{Δ} base-out prism which he will tape on his glasses. If no prescription, have the patient buy a cheap pair of sunglasses and pop out the lens. Patient will start close to the TV or picture until a *clear single image* is seen, slowly move back from TV until image blurred or doubled and again move toward the TV, once a *clear single picture* is regained start again and the objective is 6 meters. This recession practice is performed 20 minutes a day, patient is seen at four to six week intervals to monitor improvement and increase strength of prism. Surgical management is considered if a stable alignment is not achieved in six months.

iii. Surgical management can be considered without occlusion therapy or fusional amplitude training. It depends upon the amount and frequency of exodeviation and refixation with the alternate cover test.

iv. Postop Treatment

NOTE: It is important to measure in right and left fields for any incomitance.

If overcorrection is 5-20$^{\Delta}$ E (T) – ET for either distance or near or both distance and near, give no treatment but check patient at weekly or two week intervals. Deviation should gradually become less in amount and constancy at each visit. Should it stay the same or esotropia increases – initiate full time alternate occlusion to stop the over-convergence response.

The over-convergence response is due to the fact that when the patient was previously exotropic, they learned to converge to eliminate diplopia and continued to over-converge to eliminate diplopia in the new, esotropic position. The patient should be seen at one week intervals since the esotropia may be quickly resolved once the stimulus to over-convergence is eliminated.

a. Check if hyperopia is present – even one diopter of hyperoptic correction plays a significant part in eliminating the *eso*deviation.
b. If the hyperopic correction was given and the ET was resolved, follow and treat as an accommodative esotropia.
c. If a hyperopic correction has no effect, give Fresnel base-out prisms in the amount to slightly overcorrect the esodeviation. The patients should be seen at two week intervals to attempt gradual reduction of prism. The method is as follows:

   5$^{\Delta}$ BI clip-on prism is worn for 20 minutes in the office. If fusion is still maintained, a 3 to 5$^{\Delta}$ reduction in prism is prescribed. If reduction of press-on prism is unsuccessful following a two month period – surgical intervention is indicated.

v. Marked Overcorrection – 25-45$^{\Delta}$ET - Consider blind spot syndrome
   a. Usually glasses have no effect consider full time alternate occlusion to stop the over convergence impulse. Check at two week intervals if the esotropia continues to decrease.

b. If no improvement for two weeks give base-out press-on prism in the amount to slightly overcorrect the esotropia. In a fusion or no fusion response, surgery is performed for the total amount of esodeviation.

vi. Under-correction – Minimal Residual Exophoria

IMPORTANT: Remember to re-measure in all fields to observe any incomitance. No treatment indicated, but observe the patient at 3 to 4 month intervals.

vii. Marked under-correction – Residual X(T) or XT
If moderate to large exodeviation is present postop minus lenses may be considered in children as a temporizing method. However in this situation of marked under-correction, press-on prisms play significant roles to prognosticate the patient's sensory and motor response for additional surgery.

3. Convergence Insufficiency (X - X(T) – XT) – Deviation greater for near

a. Etiology: anatomic, optical, accommodative, or Neurogenic
   i. General disease or debility; e.g. toxic conditions.
   ii. Psychopathic instability.
   iii. Secondary to divergence excess.

b. Characteristics
   i. Late onset.
   ii. Asthenopia associated with near work.
   iii. X or XT greater for near, less X or ortho for distance.
   iv. Remote NPC, more remote when tested with red filter.
   v. Prism divergence normal.
   vi. Prism convergence low for distance and near.
   vii. Amblyopia rare.
   viii. NRC is usually present.
   ix. Suppression more frequent for near.
   x. Accommodation may be weak or the patient may demonstrate a low AC/A ratio or fall in the hypoaccommodative group.

c. Treatment
   i. Red filter with penlight progression to bridge of nose or NPC with an accommodative target.
   ii. Initiate base-out practice in the following situations.
      a. Red Glass progressive practice to bridge of nose.
      b. Reading or various near projects in young children.
      c. If suppression is present teach the child or adult physiologic diplopia awareness. Could use pencil or finger.

   In both situations begin with 5^{Δ} base-out loose prism and gradually increase to 20^{Δ} base-out prism (total of 20 minutes per day at five minute intervals).

   iii. If symptoms are not relieved, surgery is decided on the total amount of near deviation and in some cases, press-on prisms may be considered preoperatively to determine postop response.

4. Convergence Insufficiency and Hypoaccommodation.

   In cases where accommodation is not used [as in presbyopia, uncorrected myopia (requires no accommodation for close vision), uncorrected moderate to high hyperopia who suffers fatigue from accommodative effort], XT may develop for near. Treatment is the same as for convergence insufficiency. Care must be paid to proper correction of refractive error and this alone may be sufficient treatment in many cases. Wear correction for one month and do simple NPC exercises with a red filter and a light. If symptoms still present, attempt a trial with base-in Fresnel bifocal in the amount to neutralize deviation to check if symptoms are relieved. Once symptoms are relieved, increase relative fusional convergence and slowly reduce the base-in Fresnels. If a reduction is unsuccessful, surgery is considered as described in the above convergence insufficiency group.

B. Constant Exotropia

1. Exotropia-Basic, Divergence Excess, Convergence Insufficiency Type.

   Probably most strabismic patients in this category were originally intermittent in character and, with time, become constant. They may follow the pattern of any of the previously discussed groups or a combination of them.

   a. Treatment
      i. Proper correction of refractive error and eliminate amblyopia in children.
      ii. Measure in primary position at infinity, 6 meters, 1/3 meters, also in right-left, up-down, gazes at distance.
      iii. With neutralized prism in the office evaluate the response with the red glass and Worth 4-dot test at distance and near. Also check stereopsis.
      iv. Management and surgery depends upon type of exodeviation as discussed in the previous sections.
      v. Postop treatment (under-corrected)
         (a) Phoric or intermittent (under 10 to 15^{Δ}), increase and stabilize relative fusional convergence with loose base-out prisms. Press-on prism reduction is usually unsuccessful.
         (b) If residual exodeviation is 20^{Δ} or greater, prescribe a base-in press-on prism for 1 to 2 weeks to assess sensory and motor response. In the presence of no fusion, the patient may be acceptable cosmetically and additional surgical management may not be indicated. In a fusion response, attempt gradual reduction of base-in press-on prisms. However, if reduction is unsuccessful, additional surgery may be considered.
         (c) If residual 25^{Δ} XT or more, additional surgery is indicated. Before doing next procedure, initiate press-on prisms to determine postoperative response.
         (d) Minus lenses may be considered as a temporary management.

vi. Post-op Treatment (overcorrected group)
   (a) Initiate full-time alternate patch to stop over convergence response. Check patient at two week intervals and continue alternate occlusion until esodeviation is resolved. Discontinue occlusion if no change in esodeviation for 2 consecutive weeks and initiate press-on prism management.
   (b) Refer to section on press-on prism management in basic, divergence excess and convergence insufficiency group.

2. Sensory XT

Early infancy or after adolescence, the vision of an eye becomes grossly defective due to congenital deformity or a result of an injury. It is very probable that the affected eye will become divergent.

a. Characteristics
   i. Onset at any time.
   ii. Uniocular strabismus.
   iii. Stable angle of deviation at distance and near.

b. Treatment
   i. Occlusion Therapy – patch the dominant eye to improve VA in the defective amblyopic eye. Check types of occlusion in amblyopia lecture.
   ii. Once optimum VA is achieved in the defective vision eye, attempt to facilitate central or peripheral fusion with Fresnel press-on prisms. Press-on prism is placed in front of preferred eye (if not tolerated) transfer to the defective visual acuity eye. Treat as discussed in Press-On Prism lecture.
   iii. If fusion is present with POP, surgery can be considered with the assurance of obtaining fusion postoperatively. If no fusion response or diplopia surgery is performed for cosmesis only.

3. Consecutive XT (Also referred as secondary XT)

   a. Characteristics
      i. An accommodative ET, especially with a high AC/A ratio, may become XT due to his hyperopic correction.
      ii. An ET patient over responds to surgery and becomes an XT. A consecutive XT may develop immediately postoperatively or several weeks or months later. An over response following bimedial recessions usually shows a divergence excess type XT. An over response following a recess-resect procedure usually shows a convergence insufficiency type of deviation.

   b. Treatment
      i. Overcorrected hyperope-consecutive XT. Treatment is refractive and reduction of plus sphere correction until the patient is esophoric or under 10 prism diopters of exodeviation. Testing for the amount of cut is done with minus clip-on spheres and muscle measurements in the office. However, high hyperopes will need enough correction for good vision and, if still exotropic, a trial of base-in press-on prisms can be attempted to facilitate fusion. If *fusion present*, attempt to increase convergence amplitudes and slowly reduce the prism. If prisms cannot be reduced, surgery is performed for total amount of prisms prescribed. If no fusion present and cosmetically acceptable, further treatment is not indicated.

      ii. In *intermittent* or constant exotropia patients who have undergone two or more unsuccessful XT surgeries, *minus lens therapy* is an excellent temporizing modality to reduce the exodeviation. It provides cosmesis in exotropia (with no fusion) and comfortable SBV in X(T) fusion patients. To determine the strength of minus lenses, the patient attends a 20/30 target at six meters. The strength of minus lenses is increased at 1 diopter increments until a 20/30 target at six meters becomes blurred.

III. Incomitant Manifest Exodeviation

A. Third Cranial Nerve Palsy (Ocular Motor Nerve) - Anatomy

1. Anatomy - Primary Ocular Motor Nerve of the Eye

Originates - In front of cerebral aqueduct.

- Midbrain areas of brainstem
- Runs through the cavernous sinus
- Enters through superior orbital fissure
- Divides
  - Superior division innervates SR and eyelid levator muscle
  - Inferior division innervates the MR, IR, IO muscle
- Carries parasympathetic fibers to pupil sphincter and ciliary body muscles

Parasympathetic Nervous System

1. Part of the autonomic nervous system
2. Nerve fibers to the eye travel within the 3rd nerve and provide innervation to ciliary body for accommodation, aqueous production and sphincter to decrease pupil size (miosis).
3. Controlled by acetylcholine-chemical allows nerve transmission used by cholinesterase.

B. Characteristics and Pathologic condition

1. Sudden onset, accident, vascular or viral.
2. Onset accompanied by severe pain on ipsilateral forehead and face.
3. CT angiogram must be ordered right away to rule out aneurysm of posterior communicating artery.
4. Eye is down and out.
5. Weakness of muscles innervated by 3rd nerve.

6. Includes the eyelid levator, IO, MR, IR, SR and sometimes pupillary sphincter and ciliary muscles.
7. Involved eye deviates outward, slightly downward and droopy (ptotic) eyelid without lid fold.
8. Pupil may be dilated accommodation reduced.
9. Postures to fuse.

C. Treatment

Surgery

IV. Medial Rectus Paralysis (Rare)

A. Etiology

A partial third nerve palsy only involving the medial rectus is rare. It should be differentiated from internuclear ophthalmoplegia with an etiology of a lesion in the medial longitudinal fasciculus. With internuclear ophthalmoplegia adduction is nil unilaterally or bilaterally with asymmetric nystagmus in abduction. Myasthenia gravis also needs to be ruled out before diagnosis of medial rectus palsy is made.

B. Characteristics

1. Limitation of adduction.
2. Eyes usually abducted, but may be parallel in primary position due to convergence and active accommodative-convergence innervation.
3. Frequently associated with dysfunction of the oblique muscles.

C. Treatment

Surgery

Chapter 8

VERTICAL DEVIATIONS

I. Hyperphoria

A. Etiology

1. Abnormal attachments or insertions of vertically-acting muscles.
2. Contracture of the antagonist or yoke of originally paretic muscle which has recovered.
3. Weakness of one or more vertically-acting muscles.

B. Diagnosis (utilizing the cover/uncover test, alternate cover test with prisms)

The following measurements must be performed:

1. Distance and near
   a. If greater at distance, may be a rectus muscle involvement.
   b. If greater at near, may be an oblique muscle involvement.
2. Measure with either eye fixing to check if primary-secondary deviation is present.
3. Check for incomitance. Measure in right and left gazes, straight up and down, up to the right, down to the right, up to the left and down to the left.

C. Comitant Deviation – Hyperphoria (same distance and near)

1. Characteristics
   a. Deviation is same for distance and near and in all directions of gaze.
   b. Normal versions.
   c. Vertical deviation may or may not affect horizontal amplitudes and stereopsis.
   d. *Vertical amplitudes* may be larger than normal especially in direction opposite to that of the deviation especially in longstanding vertical deviation.

D. *Incomitant Deviation - Hyperphoria* – differs for distance and near and various direction of gazes.

1. Characteristics
   a. Greatest deviation found in field (s) of paretic muscle (s)
   b. Primary and secondary deviations may be present
   c. Versions may reveal over-and under-action of vertically-acting muscle (s)
   d. Compensatory head-tilt or face turn.
   e. Horizontal amplitudes good to poor.

E. Treatment (only symptomatic patients)

Comitant or incomitant deviation

1. Attempt to increase vertical amplitudes in the opposite direction of deviation. If a right hyperphoria, increase vertical amplitudes in the opposite direction, i.e. base-up prism amplitudes. This treatment can be performed with a penlight and red filter or physiologic diplopia awareness.
2. Horizontal amplitudes should also be improved if limited. Stable horizontal fusion helps to control the vertical component. Physiologic diplopia awareness can be used as a 'check mark'.
3. If patient is still symptomatic, give base-up or base-down press-on prisms in the amount to correct the hyper present. If there is a difference for distance and near, use the respective amounts in upper and lower segments of the lens (If no glasses worn, prescribe a pair of plano spectacles).
4. If symptoms are relieved with the press-on prisms, permanent prisms should be given. Slab-off prisms are given at near if there is a difference in distance and near measurements. In cases where the amount of hyper is too great for permanent prisms; surgery is done to correct the deviation.
5. Surgery is also recommended:
   a. With significant incomitance.
   b. To eliminate very obvious compensating head or face posture.

II. Manifest Vertical Deviations

Comitant and Incomitant

A. Comitant Hypertropia

1. Etiology
   a. Originally incomitant vertical strabismus (usually congenital which has become comitant with time).
   b. Abnormalities of insertion or attachments of vertical muscles.
   c. Asymmetry of orbit or displacement of the globe. (Hypoglobus)

2. Characteristics
   a. Frequently vertical deviation is associated with horizontal strabismus, but vertical component is the primary factor.
   b. Deviation is the same with either eye fixing and in all directions of gaze.
   c. Amblyopia or suppression frequently present.
   d. ARC may be present due to a constant angle.
   e. Compensatory head posture frequently present (retained after spread of comitance).

3. Treatment
   a. Orthoptics ineffective.
   b. *If fusion* present either on the Synoptophore or with Fresnel prisms (check monthly and gradually reduce prisms). Treat amblyopia if present in children and place Fresnel prism in front of dominant eye, non-dominant eye in adults.
   c. If reduction of prism is unsuccessful ground in prisms or surgery.
   d. If no fusion – surgery if cosmetically unacceptable.

B. Incomitant Hypertropia

1. Superior Oblique Palsy – Example (Left Superior Oblique Palsy)
   a. Etiology: Paretic in origin. Superior oblique palsy is the most commonly seen paretic vertical muscle.
   b. Causes: Vascular disease, inflammation, viral, trauma, most frequently congenital.
   c. Characteristics

i. Head-tilt most characteristic; head tilted to side opposite the paretic muscle.
ii. If head forcibly tilted to side of paralyzed eye, the eye rotates upward.
iii. OS deviated upward and deviation increases down and to the right.
iv. Main limitation of motion is down and to the right.
v. Diplopia torsional and vertical. (Separation greatest down and to the right.)

d. Tests
   i. Inspection: OS is higher, corneal light displaced downward, head-tilt to the right shoulder, chin lower.
   ii. Cover test: Covered, OS deviates upward. Covered, OD downward (greater amount). Deviation OD is greater under cover with OS fixing (secondary deviation).
   iii. Ductions: Limitation down and in.
   iv. Versions: incomitant increases in lower right field.
   v. Diplopia test: vertical separation increasing in lower field – greatest down and to the right. Red glass over OD – distal image is white, therefore LSO is lagging.
   vi. Lancaster Red-Green: patient attempts to place his green light over the examiner's red light - the green is higher in primary position. The green light is farther above the red in right 1ower field. If patient holds red light, the red is well below the green in that field. (Demonstrates primary secondary deviations). (Green OS, red OD in Lancaster Red-Green). This is a fovea to fovea test–the light goes where the light is.
   vii. Bielschowsky head tilt Test: OS is in a position of extortion since the superior oblique cannot intort. Vertical corneal meridian is adjusted by the patient tilting his head to the right shoulder. If head is forcibly tilted to the left shoulder, intorsion would occur from the action of LSO and LSR. Since LSO is paralyzed, the LSR acts alone and being mainly an elevator, elevates the left eye. This is the diagnostic test for LSO palsy.

viii. 3-Step Test for Single Paretic Muscle.
   a. Primary Position – Hyper /Hypodeviation
   b. Lateral Gazes – Deviation is greater in the gaze the paretic muscle normally functions
   c. Head Tilt – Superior – Same side
      – Inferior – Opposite side

NOTE: One problem with long-standing LSO palsy changes in other muscles occur when patient fixing with the paretic eye. A patient with an LSO palsy will show a lag of RSR on versions. LSO is paralyzed and LIO is not opposed, becomes contracted and requires less innervation. Yoke of LIO is RSR and it receives less innervation (Hering's Law) and lags in versions. This is termed Inhibitional Palsy of the Contralateral Antagonist, or more appropriately Inhibitional Palsy of Yoke of the Antagonist.

e. Treatment

Torsion may be a barrier to fusion of images and should be measured with the Double Maddox Rod Test. If torsion is under 5 ° – no barrier to fusion.

1. If patient fusing with minimal head-tilt, no symptoms and fair amplitudes, no treatment.
2. If head-tilt minimal, fusing, but has symptoms, increase and stabilize horizontal amplitudes.
3. If head-tilt marked, fusing with compensatory position, surgery is indicated.
4. If head-tilt marked, but only to avoid diplopia, no fusion with compensatory position; surgery may or may not be successful in eliminating the head tilt.

C. Greatest Field Of Action of the Vertical Muscle Using 'H' Design–Demonstrating the 3-Step Test

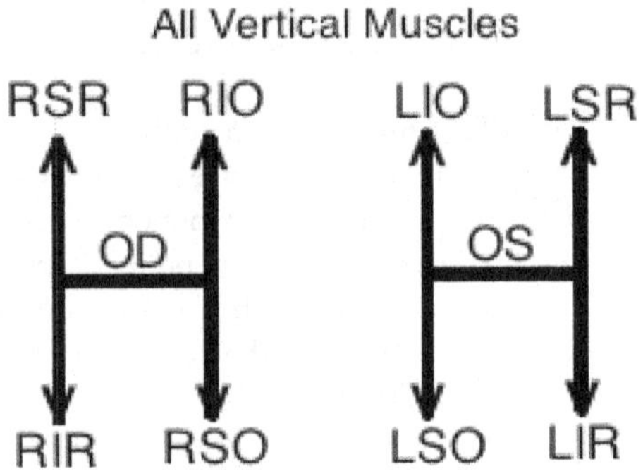

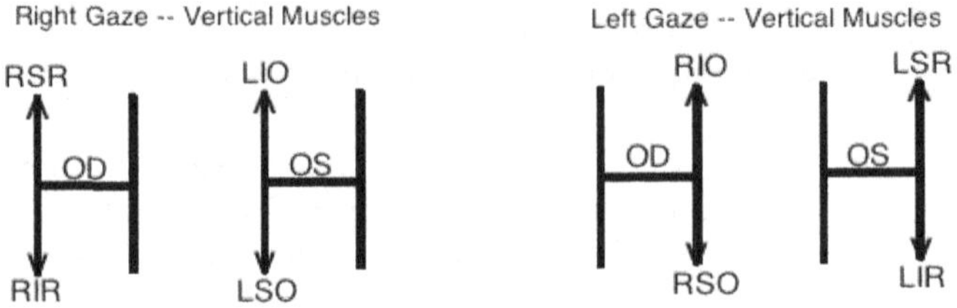

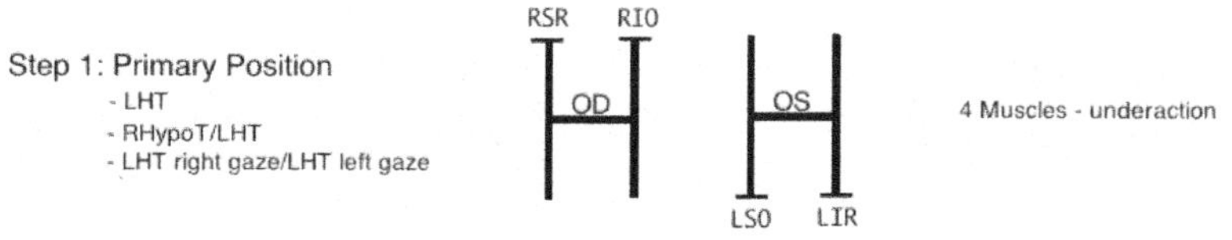

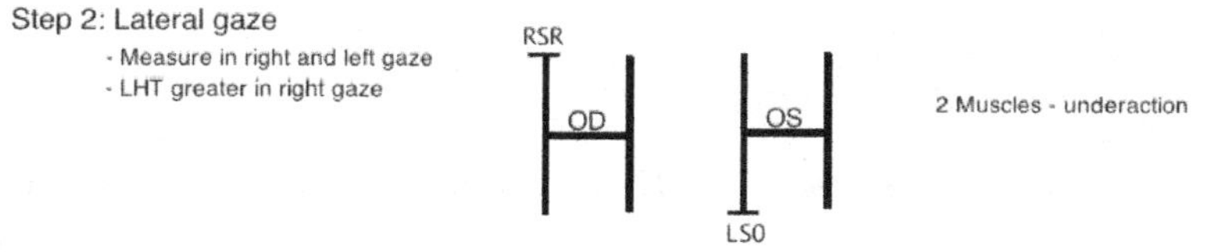

The remaining two muscles in lateral gaze will always be either:

> Two Superiors – A rectus of one eye and an oblique of the other eye.
>
> Two Inferiors – A rectus of one eye and an oblique of the other eye.

Head Tilt Theory:

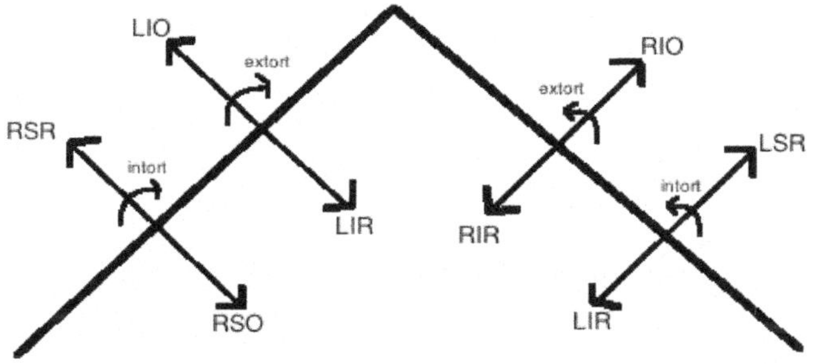

- Superiors are synergists for intorsion and antagonists for vertical movements.
- Inferiors are synergists for extorsion and antagonists for vertical movements.

Step 3: Head Tilt Test
- RSR vs LSO
- Right Tilt = RSR } underaction
- Left Tilt = LSO

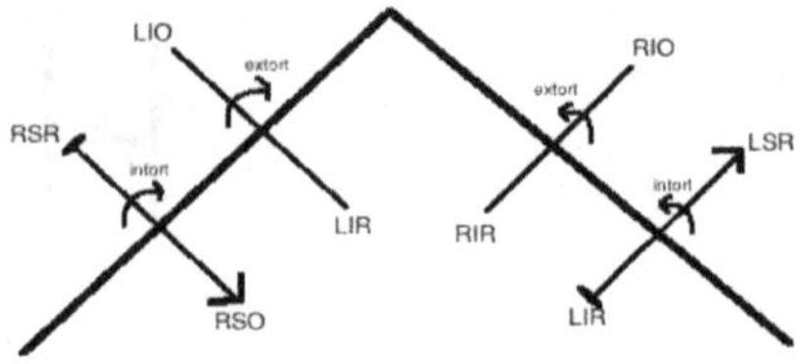

When the choice is:

Two Superiors – The tilt with the greatest vertical is to the same side as the eye with the paretic muscle.

Two Inferiors – The tilt with the greatest vertical is to the opposite side of the eye with the paretic muscle.

HINT: Head Tilt: Superiors = same side
Inferiors = opposite side

D. Three Step Test for Single Paretic Muscle Using "H" Design

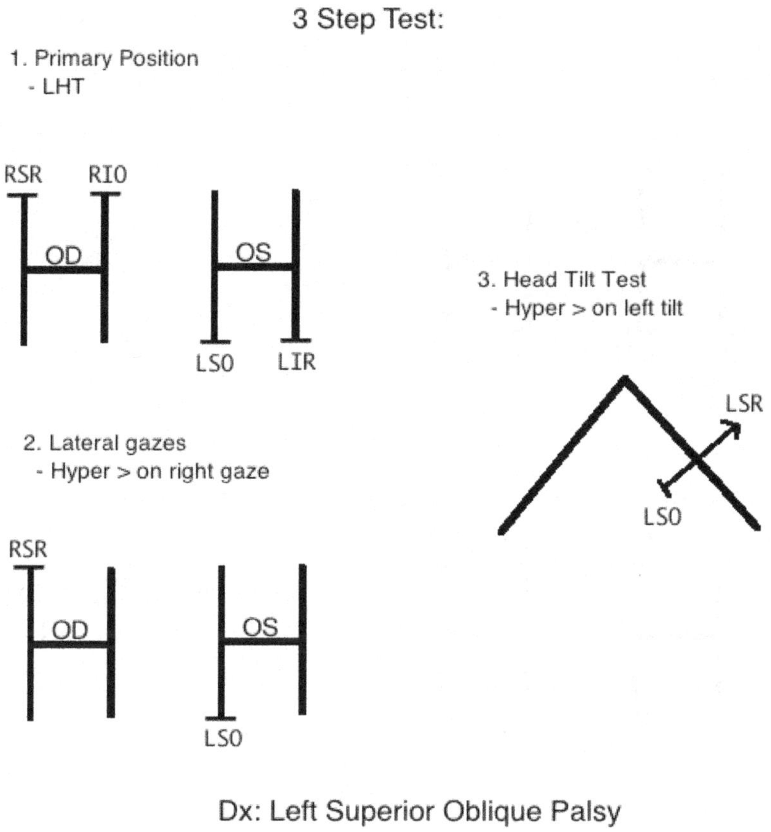

E. DX 'BISO' Palsy

3 Step Test - Bilateral SOP

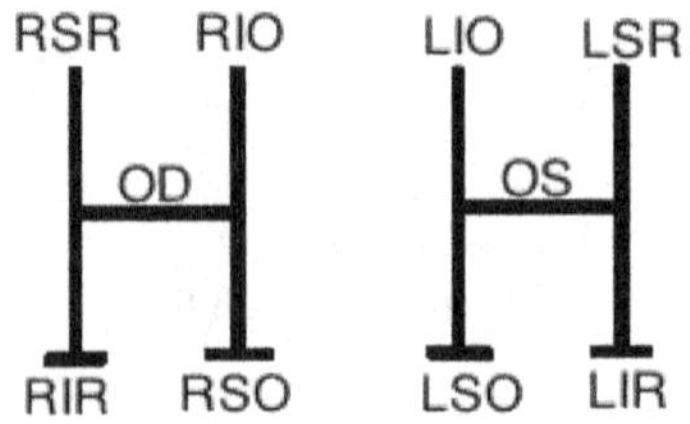

1. Primary Position
   - RHT or LHT

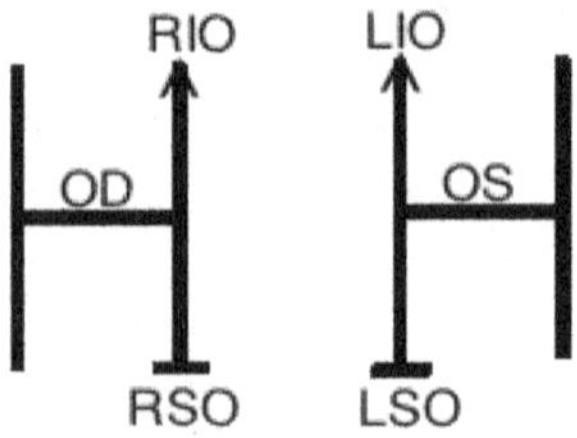

2. Lateral Gazes
   - Alternating Hypers
   - LHT <---> RHT

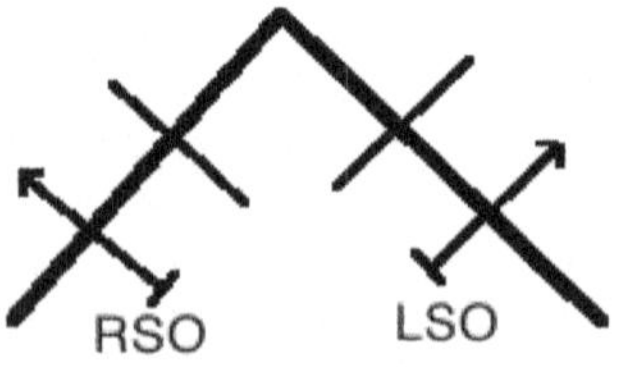

3. Head Tilt
   - + R/L
   - LHT = RHT

F. Diagnostic Test to Isolate a Vertical Muscle Palsy-With Circles (patient has left hypertropia)

3 Step Test-Circles

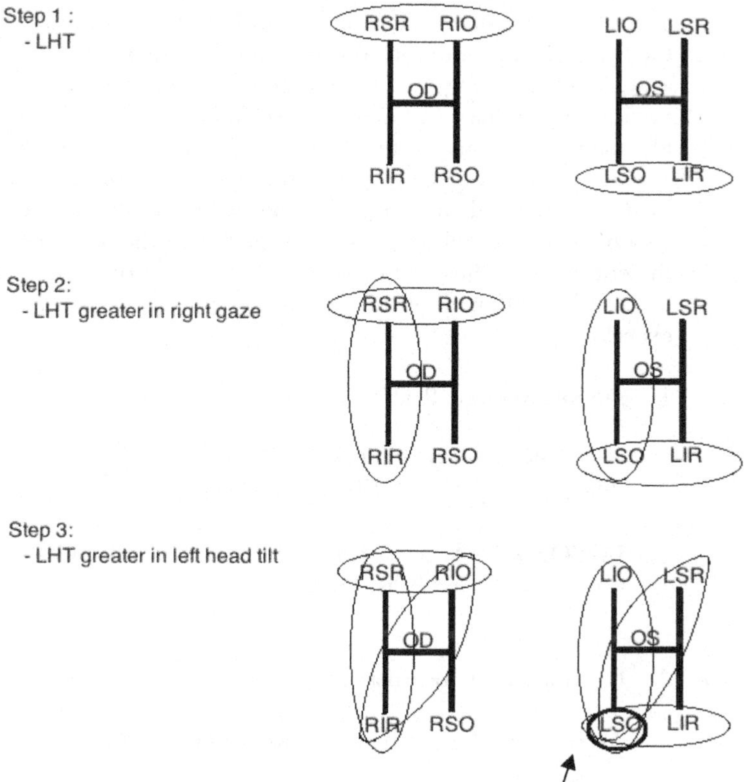

ALL THREE CIRCLES INTERSECT

Isolates to LSO Palsy

G. Double Maddox Rod Test Evaluate Ex/In Cyclotorsion

For quantitative determination of a cyclodeviation, red and white Maddox rods are placed in a trial frame, the red before the right and the white before the left eye. The direction of the glass rods is aligned with the 90° marks of the trial frame. A small scratch on the metal frame of the Maddox rods facilitates this alignment. Special care must be taken to avoid tilting the trial frames during the test. The patient looks through the Maddox rods and is shown a penlight, the images of which appear as horizontal streaks. A vertical prism may be added to separate the images for easier identification. If one of the lines (say, the red one) appears slanted toward the nose excyclotropia of the right eye is present. The red Maddox rod is then turned by the ophthalmologist (or by the patient) until the red line is seen parallel with the white line. If at the end of this adjustment the scratched mark points for example, toward the 100° mark of the right trial frame, the patient has a right excyclotropia of 10°.

1. Double Maddox Rod Test

   LSO Palsy – Extorsion OS
   Bilateral SO palsy – Bilateral excyclotorsion

   IMPORTANT: If 15° torsion bilateral superior oblique palsy is present. (Daryl Ellis, M.D.)

2. Hemifacial Microsomia in SO palsy

   Asymmetric Facial Changes Associated With Ocular Torticollis

   Patients with multiple types of torticollis including face turns, show similar appearance of facial compression on side of the torticollis, the tilt or turn itself cause the asymmetry. Head tilts are frequently associated with nasal tip deviation to the side of the torticollis in SO palsy.

DOUBLE MADDOX ROD TEST

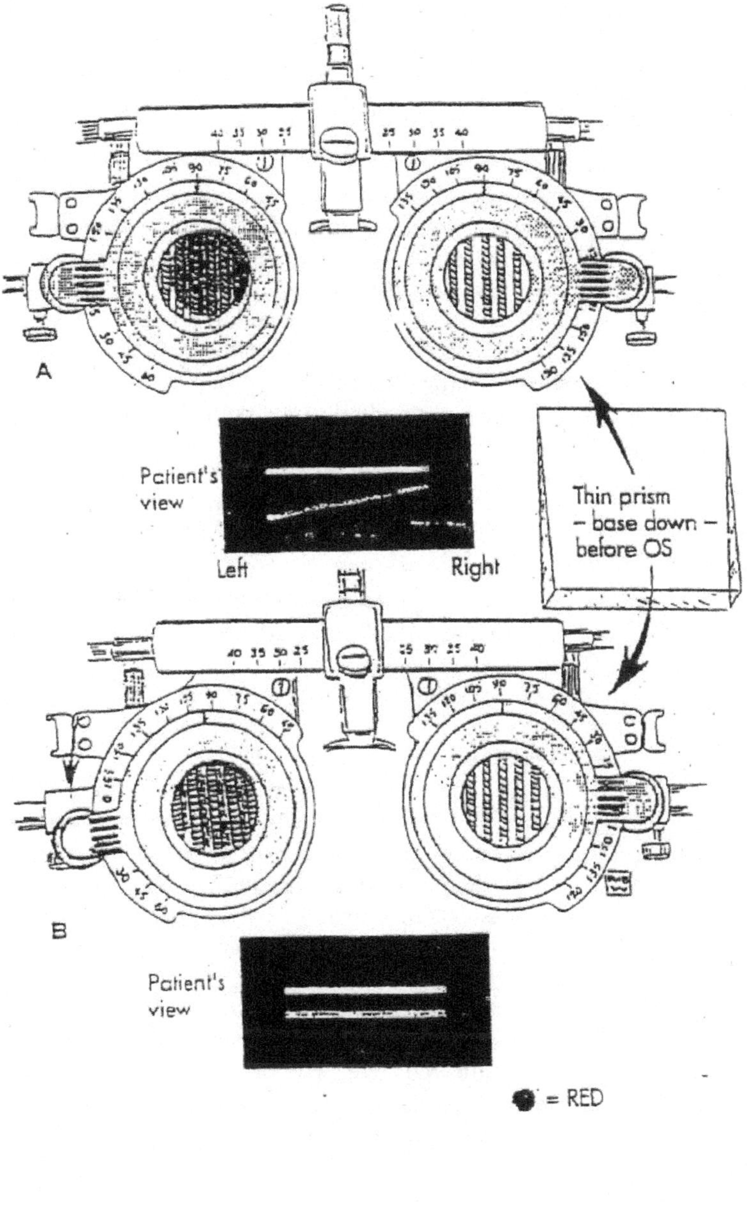

3. Inferior Oblique Palsy (Example: Right Inferior Oblique Palsy)

   Much less common than that of SO; less annoying to the patient since it involves the upper fields more than the lower fields.

   a. Characteristics
      i. Downward deviation of OD.
      ii. Angle of squint increases looking up and to the left.
      iii. Deviation OS under cover greater when OD fixing (secondary deviation).
      iv. Limitation of rotation up and to the left.
      v. Vertical diplopia --Image of the right eye is above the image of the left eye.
      vi. Head elevated, tilted to the right shoulder.

   b. Tests
      Inspection -- OD lower, corneal reflex displaced upward OD. Chin up, head-tilt to the right shoulder.

      i. Cover Test: OD covered, it turns down. Shift cover to OS, marked upward deviation behind cover (secondary deviation).
      ii. Ductions: limitation OD up and in.
      iii. Versions: incomitance increases in left upper field.
      iv. Diplopia test with red glass: vertical separation of image increases in upper fields. This indicates paralysis of an elevator muscle. Separation of images greatest up and to the left, the distal image red over OD*)*, therefore RIO is lagging.
      v. Lancaster Red-Green: (the light goes where the eye is) When patient attempts to place green light over red the green light is projected much higher in primary position (secondary deviation). The green light is farther above the red in left upper field. When patient holds the red light, it is below the green in the same field of gaze, but less separated in primary position. (Green OS, red OD in Lancaster Red-Green).

vi. Three Step Test
   (a) Left hypertropia in primary position.
   (b) Greater in left gaze.
   (c) Greater vertical deviation with left head tilt.

vii. Bielschowsky Test: Since RIO normally extorts, in paralysis, the vertical corneal meridian turns inward. This is adjusted with head tilted to the right. If head forcibly tilted to the left, compensation by extorsion of OD would result from RIO, RIR. Since RIO paralyzed, RIR pulls the eye down due to its main action of depression.

c. Treatment – Surgery

4. Superior Rectus Palsy (Example: Left Superior Rectus Palsy)

May be congenital and associated with ptosis of upper lid.

a. Characteristics
   i. OS deviated downward.
   ii. Vertical deviation increases looking up and to the left.
   iii. Upward deviation OD under cover greater than left hypo under cover (secondary deviation).
   iv. Limitation is greater up and to the left.
   v. Diplopia – vertical - as image higher. Vertical separation is greater up and to the left.
   vi. Seldom any head-tilt.

b. Tests
   Inspection - OS lower, corneal reflex displaced upward -- chin raised, rare head-tilt to right shoulder.

   i. Cover Test: covered OS deviated downward; when OD is covered, it turns upward with greater vertical deviation (secondary deviation).
   ii. Ductions: limitation of movement up and out.
   iii. Versions: incomitance increases in upper left field.
   iv. Diplopia Test: vertical separation of images increasing in upper fields. Indicates paralysis of elevators. Separation of images greatest up and left. Distal image is white (red glass over OD). Therefore LSR is lagging.

v. Lancaster Red-Green: patient attempts to place green over red, the green is lower in the primary position. Green light farther below in left upper field. Patient holds red, the red is farthest above green in upper left field. (secondary deviation). (Green OS, red OD in Lancaster Red-Green).

vi. Three-step test
   (a) RHT in primary position
   (b) Greater deviation looking to the left
   (c) Greater vertical measurements with head tilted to left shoulder

c. Treatment - Surgery

5. Inferior Rectus Palsy (Example: Right Inferior Rectus Palsy)

More annoying paralysis in fresh case than SR involvement because lower reading field is involved.

a. Characteristics
   i. Right eye deviated upward.
   ii. Angle of deviation increases down and right.
   iii. Deviation of as under cover greater than OD under cover (secondary deviation).
   iv. Limitation of movement in OD down and to the right in the involved eve.
   v. Diplopia - vertical, image of OD lower, with greatest separation down and to the right.
   vi. Slight head-tilt to right.

b. Tests

Inspection -- OD appears higher, corneal reflection displaced downward. Head tilted to right shoulder, chin lowered.

   i. Cover Test: OD covered, deviated upward; when OS covered, deviates downward in a greater amount (secondary deviation).
   ii. Versions: incomitance increases in lower right field.
   iii. Diplopia Test: vertical separation of images is greater in lower fields (indicates paralysis of depressor muscle). Sensation of image greatest down and right. Distal image is red (red OD). Therefore, RIR is lagging.

iv. Lancaster Red-Green: patient attempts to place his green light over the red, green is lower in primary position. Green is farther below in 1ower right field (secondary deviation). Patient holds red, red is above green in lower right field, but less distance away (primary deviation). (Green OS, red OD in Lancaster Red-Green).

v. Three Step Test
   (a) RHT in primary position
   (b) Greater deviation in right gaze
   (c) Greater vertical deviation with left head tilt

c. Treatment - Surgery

III. Double Hypertropia

A. Etiology

Paresis of similar acting vertical muscles in both eyes. If both muscles are equally paretic, the amount of right and left hyper will be equal; if not, the vertical deviation will be greater when fixing with the eye with the greater involvement. Direction of hyper may change depending which eye is fixing or in the different direction of gaze.

B. Treatment – vertical prisms or surgery

IV. Dissociated Vertical Divergence DVD

A. What is DVD?

Spontaneous slow upward drift associated with abduction and extorsion of the affected eye. The deviated eye extorts during its ascent then intorts as it descended to resume fixation. Becomes manifest when binocular vision input is disrupted mechanically, optically or sensorially.

B. DVD was a term introduced by Bielschowsky in 1943.
Synonyms:
1. Alternating sursumduction – ASD
2. As occlusion hypertropia
3. Anaphoria
4. Dissociated hyperphoria
5. Double hyperphoria

C. Etiology

1. Abnormal excitation of the vertical divergence center (Jampolsky 1986)[4]
2. Abnormally in the development of normal centers (Harcourt, et al 1980)[5]
3. A compensated mechanism to dampen cyclovertical latent nystagmus (Guyton 1998)[6]
4. Recapitulates the primitive Dorsal light reflex which asymmetrical visual input to the 2 eyes evokes a vertical divergence movement of the eyes (Brodsky 2002)[7]

D. Characteristics (May be present in one or both eyes)

1. Either eye makes a slow and irregular drift upward under cover which is usually accompanied with some extorsion. When cover is removed, the eye intorts as it drifts down slowly.
2. In changing fixation from one to the other eye, one does not observe an upward movement of one eye by a downward movement of the other as seen in vertical deviations. In DVD, the non-fixing eye consistently drifts upward.
3. DVD occurs in other cardinal positions of gaze as well as in primary position,
4. It may be present in binocular fixation which is called "pure" DVD and only becomes manifest when one eye is occluded or under fatigue and stress. In these individuals, the vertical amplitudes in both directions are higher than in patients found without DVD.
5. Most commonly found superimposed upon a horizontal or vertical deviation or both.
6. VA in both eyes may be normal, but if amblyopia is present, dissociation occurs more readily in the amblyopic eye.
7. Diplopia is usually not present in patients with DVD. Suppression of the deviating eye occurs readily (Bielschowsky emphasized the high incidence of DVD in patients with either congenital or acquired amblyopia.)
8. Nystagmus and DVD frequently co-exist; Billet and Ehrlich stated that latent nystagmus is found in every case of DVD and in fact induces DVD.
9. Vertical amplitudes are variable.
10. First noted two to five years of age.
11. Presence of a manifest head tilt in 35% of patients.

E. Distinguishing Features of DVD and Inferior Oblique (IO) Overaction[8]

DVD	IO Overaction
1. Elevation in adduction and abduction	1. Elevation only in adduction
2. Comitant in fields of gaze	2. Incomitant in action IO
3. Variable hyper	3. Not variable
4. No A or V pattern	4. Normally associated 'V' pattern
5. Same hyper up and down gaze	5. More hyper up than down gaze
6. No hypotropia in corresponding opposite eye	6. Corresponding hypotropia in the opposite eye
7. May co-exist with IO Overaction	7. IO overaction always present
8. Frequently associated with infantile ET and congenital nystagmus	8. Not associated

F. Method of Measuring DVD:

Step 1. Concurrent horizontal deviation is neutralized first with prism alternate cover test.

Step 2. Amount of vertical deviation is measured by placing base down prism in front of the eye with DVD.

Step 3. The amount of base down prism is increased until no downward movement is seen; the induced hypotropia in the opposite eye is ignored.

Step 4. In presence of a co-existing, true hypertropia (corresponding hypotropia in the opposite eye).

- Amount is measured by increasing base down prism in front of the DVD eye, while observing diminishing hypotropia shift in the fellow eye upon alternate cover test.

- After the full amount of corresponding hypotropia is neutralized, the additional hypertropia measurement is due to DVD.

G. Associated with Manifest Head Tilt

- A manifested head tilt with DVD may be present in patients with or without fixation preference, prior vertical muscle surgery.

- In patients with fixation preference, in some case the angle of deviation increased with a forced head tilt to the contralateral side of DVD and decreases with a forced head tilt to the ipsilateral side.

- With alternate fixation the angle of deviation is the same with right and left head tilt.

- Atypical responses are not influenced by oblique overaction.

- The size and control of DVD is measured in both the natural (if manifested head tilt is present) and forced primary head position and after forced head position to the right and left.

H. Bielschowsky Phenomenon

This phenomenon is an interesting characteristic of DVD. The amplitude of vertical deviation is related to the asymmetry of visual input in the 2 eyes. This effect is clearly shown by the Bielschowsky Phenomenon.

Method 1. Red filters of increment density is placed before the fixing eye causes the hypertropic eye to gradually descend even to the hypotropic position.

Method 2. Place a dark red wedge occluder before the fixing eye while the hypertropic eye is occluded. As the field of the fixing eye darkens, the occluded eye moves downward.

I. Treatment for DVD

Orthoptic Management

- Eliminate amblyopia
- Increase horizontal amplitudes
- Base down ground-in prisms in front of DVD eye

J. Surgical Management – moderate to a large DVD or the presence of manifested head tilt.
(OA-SR-IO)

V. Dissociated Horizontal Deviation DHD

A. DVD includes movements in both the horizontal and vertical planes. When the horizontal component of DVD is very prominent, the horizontal dissociation movement is labeled DHD.

B. DHD is defined as an asymmetric or unilateral slow outward deviation associated with vertical and torsional dissociated movements that can be manifest or latent. DHD is nonparalytic and does not obey Hering's law of equal innervation.

C. Distinguishing Features of DHD

1. Unilaterally or asymmetry of the exodeviation between the 2 eyes.
2. Variability and difficulty in obtaining a clear end point with prism neutralization.
3. Often times, prism neutralization produces an esodeviation in the fellow eye. This similar pattern could be produced by a paralytic strabismus in the form of primary and secondary deviation. However, no weakness in ductions, versions and incomitance is present in DHD.
4. Uncorrected refractive error can produce a pseudo DHD. An exodeviation decreases when a patient fixes with a unilateral uncorrected hyperopic eye stimulating accommodation with convergence.
5. Bielschowsky phenomenon is demonstrated in the horizontal plane. Place a darkening wedge in front of fixing eye, and the outwardly drifted eye will return and cross the midline line.

D. Three Criteria Required for True DHD

1. Minimum difference 5 Δ in amount of exodeviation when alternately fixing.
2. No limitation in ocular motility that may produce primary and secondary deviation.
3. No uncorrected anisometropia that may produce incomitance with alternate fixation.

VI. Double Elevator Palsy

This is a lack of elevation of one eye due to a weakness of both the superior rectus and the inferior oblique. The two muscles may be affected equally, but often the paralysis is more pronounced in the inferior oblique than the superior rectus. The forced duction test will differentiate it from a fibrosis of the inferior rectus. Etiology may be a unilateral supranuclear lesion.

A. Characteristics

1. Pseudo-ptosis secondary to hypotropia in opposite eye. A ptosis may also occur.
2. Marked hypertropia when fixing with the paretic eye.
3. Head-tilt directly back and a head tilt in opposite direction.
4. Phoria is intermittent in down gaze with usually good fusion and stereopsis.
5. Check if Bells is normal – if not could be due to a mechanical restriction.

B. Treatment – Surgery

VII. Brown's SO Tendon Sheath Syndrome

Etiology: Short anterior tendon sheath of SO which normally acts as a check ligament for the IO on the same side.

A. Characteristics

1. Good visual acuity OU.
2. Primary position -- hypotropia in the affected eye or no vertical deviation present.
3. Absence or gross limitation of elevation in nasal field (simulates an IO paralysis). In most cases elevation in nasal field is limited to a few degrees below the mid-horizontal plane.

4. Limitation of elevation decreases as involved eye is abducted. Full elevation with involved eye completely abducted – may demonstrate V pattern.
5. 'Downshoot' of depression of affected eye on adduction.
6. Widening of palpebral fissure on adduction of affected eye.
7. Normal excursions of involved eye in temporal field of gaze.
8. No vertical imbalance in lower field.
9. Little or no overaction of SO (no secondary contracture).
10. Backward head-tilt often present.
11. Usually good fusion and stereopsis at near.

B. Treatment – Surgery.

Chapter 9

A–V SYNDROME OR PATTERNS

I. Introduction

A or V patterns are present when there is a significant difference in the size of the deviation between up and down gazes.

A. Designations

1. A-Patterns
   a. A-Eso. The esodeviation is greater in up gaze.
   b. A-Exo. The exodeviation is greater in down gaze.
2. V-Patterns
   a. V-Eso. The esodeviation is greater in down gaze.
   b. V-Exo. The exodeviation is greater in up gaze.

B. Norms

A significant difference is 10 prism diopters for an A-pattern and 15 prism diopters for a V-pattern. When the deviation is greater in down gaze, the anomaly is worse from a therapeutic point of view because down gaze is used more than up gaze. Consequently, it is particularly important to diagnose a V-eso or A-exodeviation since the V-exo and A-eso are physiologically less disturbing.

II. Etiology

A. Obliques

There are three theories or schools of thought regarding etiology. Jampolsky, Costenbader and Parks hold that the additional horizontal deviation on vertical gaze is attributed to the abduction from the obliques.

1. V-Patterns with OAIO
   If there is an overaction of the inferior obliques, there is also excessive abduction from the inferior obliques causing less eso and more exo in up gaze.

2. A-Patterns with OASO
   If there is overaction of the superior obliques, there is also excessive abduction from the superior obliques on down gaze causing less eso and more exo on down gaze.

B. Horizontal Recti

The second school states that horizontals cause A-V patterns; lateral and medial recti being implicated (Urist). There is some evidence of supranuclear overaction of lateral rectus in upward gaze and overaction of the medial rectus in down gaze.

Use the acronym MALE to remember that Medials are shifted toward the Apex and Laterals toward the Empty space.

C. Vertical Recti

The third group implies that vertical recti are responsible. Miller claims overaction of the inferior rectus may cause V-exo or V-eso and overaction of the superior rectus can cause A-eso or A-exo.

III. Surgery

A. A-Eso

1. Significant overaction of SO.
   a. Tenotomy SO, OU.
   b. In addition to horizontal surgery with a mark A pattern.
2. No SO overaction
   a. MR surgery – raise insertion.
   b. LR surgery -lower insertion.

B. A-Exo

1. If significant SO overaction.
   a. Tenotomy SO, OU.
   b. In addition to horizontal surgery with a mark A pattern.

2. No SO overaction.
   a. MR surgery - raise insertion.
   b. LR surgery - lower insertion.

C. V-Eso

1. Significant IO overaction.
    a. Myotomy IO, OU or recession IO, OU.
    b. In addition to horizontal surgery with a mark V pattern.
2. No oblique overaction.
    a. MR surgery and lower insertion.
    b. LR surgery and raise insertion.

D. V-Exo

1. Significant IO overaction.
    a. Myotomy IO, OU or recession IO, OU.
    b. In addition to horizontal surgery with a mark V pattern.

2. No oblique overaction.
    a. MR surgery and lower insertion.
    b. LR surgery and raise insertion.

Chapter 10

CYCLODEVIATIONS

I. Definitions

A. Cyclophoria - a latent torsional deviation in which the superior pole of the vertical meridian of the cornea of one eye tips nasally (incyclophoria) or temporally (excyclophoria).

B. Cyclotropia - a manifest torsional strabismus in which the superior pole of the vertical corneal meridian of one eye tips nasally (incyclotropia) or the superior pole of the vertical corneal meridian tips temporally (excyclotropia) around the anterior-posterior axis when fusion is suspended.

NOTE: The prefixes *incyclo* and *excyclo* refer to the position of the superior pole of the vertical meridian of the cornea, *not the inclination of the image.*

II. Classification

A. Cyclophoria - may be comitant or incomitant.

B. Cyclotropia - may be constant or intermittent, comitant or incomitant.

III. Etiology

A. Optical - resulting from uncorrected or recently corrected oblique astigmatism.

B. Anatomical – abnormalities of insertion or check ligaments of the vertical muscles; paresis or overaction of the vertical muscles.

C. Innervational abnormalities.

IV. Symptoms

A. Headaches.

B. Nervous, upset, nausea, vomiting.

C. Apparent distortion and/or tilting of objects.

D. Near work may accentuate symptoms.

E. Torsional diplopia (with cyclotropia).

F. Head tilt - objective sign.

V. Tests for Determination and Measurement of Cyclodeviation

A. Maddox double prism

1. Maddox double prism is placed horizontally in a trial frame is placed before the fixing eye while the patient's attention is directed to a horizontal line drawn on a card.

2. In the presence of a cycle-deviation a tipping of the middle horizontal line (seen by the non-fixing eye) will be seen between two parallel horizontal lines (seen by the fixing eye); tipping of the center line nasally indicates extorsion of the eye; tipping temporally indicates intorsion of the eye.

Example: Maddox double prism in front of O.D.

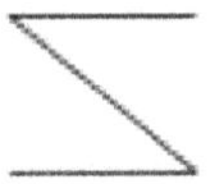

excyclodeviation O.S.
(image is incyclo-rotated)

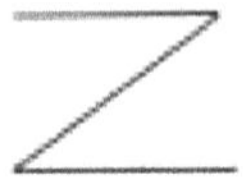

incyclodeviation O.S.
(image is excyclo-rotated)

3. The amount of deviation present can be measured by the degree of rotation of the prism required to attain parallelism of the three lines.

4. Test with each eye fixing.

B. Double Maddox Rod

1. Two Maddox rods are placed in trial frame (one red, one white). The patient's attention is directed to a light source.

2. If fusion is present, must be suspended by introduction of appropriate prism to separate the two images.

3. In the presence of a cyclodeviation the rod before the eye which sees the tilted image is rotated until parallelism of the streaks is achieved and alignment with the floor. This is a measure of the torsion present.

C. Major amblyoscope

1. Using grade one dissimilar targets, e.g., lion and cage, have patient fixate the lion. The slide presented to the non-fixing eye must contain a definite horizontal line. If the cage appears tilted, a cyclodeviation is present. The tilt of the image is in the opposite direction to the tilt of the eye.

Example: Tilting of image of the right eye

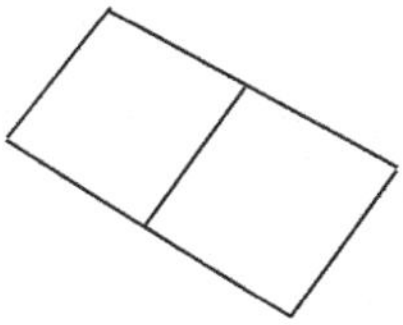

Incyclodeviation (image O.D. is extorted)

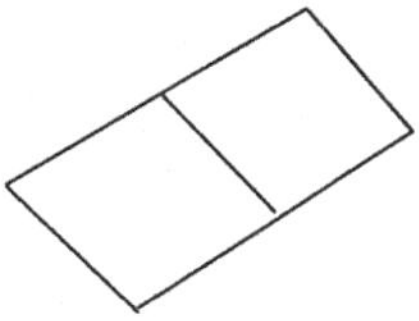

excyclodeviation (image O.D. is intorted)

2. To correct for incyclodeviation tilt the top of the slide carrier toward the patient until cage appears level. To correct for excyclodeviation tilt top of slide carrier away from the patient. The amount of deviation is read from the scale on the slide carrier arm.

3. Repeat procedure fixing the other eye.

D. Lancaster red-green test - Cyclodeviations may be diagnosed by this test but not quantitatively measured.

VI. Treatment

A. Correction of refractive error.

B. Correction of any associated vertical deviation (in phoria cases the effort to overcome the hyperphoria may accentuate the cyclophoria).

C. In an attempt to increase torsional fusional amplitudes, the cyclodeviation may be gradually increased in the opposite direction on the major synoptophore while the patient maintains fusion on the targets presented.

D. Surgical management if torsion is greater than 5 degrees with Double Maddox.

Chapter 11

PRESS-ON PRISM MANAGEMENT FOR HORIZONTAL DEVIATIONS IN CHILDREN AND ADULTS

I. Press-On Prism Management in Esotropic Children and Adults

A. Method:

1. Measure the deviation to reversal and subtract 2 diopters.
2. Measure distance and near.
3. Measure up, down, right, and left gaze.

B. Perform the following sensory test with the neutralized prism:

1. Red glass and light (distance and near).
2. Worth four dot (distance and near).
3. Stereopsis at near.

C. Place the selected press-on prism in front of the preferred eye in children and in front of the non-preferred eye in adults.

II. Esodeviation – No Previous Surgery

A. *Fusion* – two options of treatment

1. Surgery to align eyes for the total amount of esodeviation.
2. Press-on prisms can be considered preoperatively in small angle esotropia to determine response to prism alignment.
   a. 15 prism diopters or less – attempt to gradually reduce BO prism at 3-5 diopter increments. Check at one to two week intervals. If unsuccessful after three weeks, surgical management is encouraged.
   b. In patients (usually adults) who do not prefer surgery – Press-on prisms are an excellent tool in determining the correct amount of ground-in prism. Inform the patient that ground-in prisms increase with the passage of time.

NOTE: Press-on prisms over the dominant eye in children and non-preferred eye in adults.

B. No fusion - No diplopia

1. Esotropia 15 PD or greater
   a. Surgical management – if the alignment is not acceptable cosmetically.
   b. Press-on prism may be considered preoperatively in some cases to verify if good alignment is achieved with no change in sensory response.

C. *No fusion – Constant diplopia* (mainly in adult patients)

1. If binocular diplopia cannot be eliminated with prisms or blurring the deviated eye with Bangerter Foils, consider the following method utilizing a Bangerter Foil in combination with base-out prisms in front of the deviated eye.
   a. First, select the foil that made the second image least disturbing.
   b. Next, slowly increase base-out prism in front of the deviated eye to move the second image more peripherally to eliminate the awareness of diplopia.
   c. The press-on prism is place on the back side of the lens and the foil is placed on the front side of the lens and worn 2-3 weeks before prescribing a ground-in prism.
   d. If the second image has continued to remain least disturbing and the alignment is acceptable, either prescribe ground-in prisms or surgical management to align the eyes.

2. Other methods of treatment to eliminate constant intractable diplopia are:
   a. Blenderm (surgical tape)
   b. Clear contact paper
   c. Satin Scotch tape (Guyton)
   d. In patients with dragged foveal syndrome (Guyton) a Bangerter foil is placed on the front side of the lens of the deviated eye to induce a scotoma. An alternate cover test is performed to eliminate the tropia so the second vertical image is placed into the scotoma of the deviated eye. (Iacobucci, Archer and Furr)

NOTE: Surgery depends on cosmetic appearance.

III. Post ET Surgery

- Over-corrected XT – now secondary ET
- Residual ET after ET surgery

A. Check sensory and motor response with neutralized prism in the office:

1. Red Glass and light (distance and near)
2. Worth Four Dot (distance and near)
3. Stereopsis (near)

B. Sensory Response to Prisms:

1. *Fusion* - Replace selected loose prism with the press-on prism and check the patient in one to two weeks to determine if the deviation is stable and comfortable fusion is present. If fusion is still unstable at the return visit, increase the strength of the prism and check the patient at one to two week intervals until stable alignment is maintained. Surgery will be determined on the total amount of press-on prism prescribed to achieve comfortable binocular single vision.
2. *No Fusion, no diplopia, and poor cosmesis* – Before considering a second surgery, initiate press-on prism management as described in the Fusion group but the objective is to determine a cosmetically acceptable alignment to prevent a third surgery.
3. *No Fusion* – Constant diplopia (usually in adult patients), use the same procedure as discussed in "No Previous Surgery" section C.

IV. Press-On Prism Management in Exotropic Children and Adults

A. Method:

1. Measure the deviation to reversal and subtract 2 diopters.
2. Measure distance and near.
3. Measure up, down, right, and left gaze.

B. Perform the following sensory test with the neutralized prism:

1. Red glass and light (distance and near)
2. Worth four dot (distance and near)
3. Stereopsis at near

V. Exodeviation – No Previous Surgery

A. *Fusion* – Surgery

1. In children, surgery depends on refixation recovery in free space with the cover test and the frequency and length of time the exodeviation is present.
2. Occlusion of the dominant eye if amblyopia is present or alternate occlusion may be used to overcome suppression if the misalignment is observed less than 25% of the day. Patient is observed at two month intervals, if stable fusion is not obtained in 6 months, surgical management is advised.

B. *No Fusion, no diplopia* – Surgical management depends on cosmesis.

C. *No Fusion, with diplopia* (usually adults)– manage as discussed in "Esodeviation – No Previous Surgery" section C. Prisms will be oriented base-in for exodeviations.

VI. Post XT Surgery

- Over-corrected ET – now secondary XT.
- Residual XT after XT surgery.
- Check sensory and motor response with neutralized prism in the office.

A. Central Fusion – 15 PD or less:

Initiate BI press-on prism and attempt to reduce prism in 3-5 prism diopter increments. If unsuccessful after two to four weeks, use ground-in prisms or advise surgical intervention.

B. Central Fusion – 20 PD or greater:

Use press-on prism for the total amount of the exodeviation. Check patient in one to two weeks; if good alignment is maintained, plan surgery. If alignment is still unstable, give additional prism. Monitor at one to two week intervals until alignment is stable. Surgery is determined on the full amount of prism prescribed.

C. No Fusion – No diplopia:

Surgery if cosmetic appearance is not acceptable. In this group, press-on prisms are used to prognosticate if good alignment will be achieved. This prevents a third surgery.

D. No Fusion – Diplopia (usually adults):

If binocular diplopia cannot be eliminated with prisms or blurring the deviated eye with Bangerter Foils, consider the following method utilizing a Bangerter Foil in combination with base-in prisms in front of the deviated eye.

1. First, select the foil that made the second image least disturbing.
2. Next, slowly increase base-in or out prism to move the second image more peripherally to eliminate the awareness of diplopia.
3. The press-on prism is place on the back side of the lens and the foil is placed on the front side of the lens.

VII. Neurogenic and Myogenic Deviations (Recent Onset)

A. Paretic

1. Prism is preferred over patch – place in front of non-preferred eye to prevent secondary muscle contraction.
2. Residual face turn – may be present once comfortable binocular vision is achieved with press-on prism.
3. Prism reduction as the paresis slowly resolves or surgical management after six months.

B. Thyroid – Graves Eye Disease (GED).

1. Eye signs in patients with excessive hormone concentration includes: eyelid retraction, lid lag in down gaze, dry cornea, ptosis, strabismus due to fibrotic extraocular muscles and optic neuropathy. These patients have severe diplopia because the misalignment can be horizontal, vertical, or both.
2. Treatment may require multiple visits and complex surgical procedures.
   a. Medical management with a neuro-ophthalmologist.

b. Plastic surgeon to perform decompression surgery to remove the bone and scar tissue behind the eye in order to create more space for the thickened muscles and tissue.
c. Orthoptist for measurements and prism management.
d. Pediatric ophthalmologist who specializes in adult strabismus, to surgically correct eye misalignment.

3. In the majority of cases, the patient is given an eye patch to be worn in front of the affected eye (if both eyes are involved then the most affected eye) to prevent secondary contractures. This method is not cosmetically accepted by patients and prevents binocular vision. The press-on prism over the affected eye is an excellent alternative, which is not only cosmetically acceptable but facilitates binocular single vision.

4. The ocular misalignment is measured with a cover test to select the correct press-on prism to eliminate diplopia. The prism is placed on the back surface of the lens in front of the involved eye. The patient is seen at four to six week intervals during their surgical and medical management and the press-on prisms may be continually adjusted during this period.

C. Myasthenia Gravis

1. Medications – Mestinon, steroids, Cellcept.
2. Abnormality of the nerve in the muscle junction, leading to excessive muscle fatigue.
3. Eye signs include ptosis and diplopia which appear or worsens as the day progresses.
4. A trial of press-on prisms in front of the non-preferred eye may be extremely beneficial to facilitate comfortable binocular vision. These patients are very challenging because their deviations frequently change therefore it is difficult to obtain the correct prism to eliminate their diplopia.
5. If the amount of deviation is too great for ground-in prism, surgical management is advised.

VIII. Selection of the Press-On Prism, Cutting Technique, and Applying to Lens

A. Prism Placement:

1. Non-preferred eye for adults.

2. Dominant eye in children.
3. Equal OU – poorly accepted.

B. Strength and Direction of Press-On Prism:

Tests with loose prisms
1. Cover Test
2. Single Maddox
3. Red Filter
4. Diplopia in Free Space

C. Cutting Technique

1. Make sure the flat side of the prism is placed on the inside of the lens.
2. Trace the size of the lens onto the prism with a washable marker.
3. Cut prism on the line you traced so that the prism is the same size as the lens, this allows the prism to be less visible to others.

D. Applying Prism to Lens

1. Once prism is cut to size, wash prism with soapy water and rinse.
2. Place a pool of water on the inside of the lens.
3. Place prism on the pool of water and apply pressure to remove all excess water.
4. Dry lens with a cloth that is lint-free to avoid lint getting stuck in ridges of prism.
5. Advise patient how to clean and apply prism at home.

Chapter 12

EYE PRACTICES

I. Fixation and Antisuppression Practices

A. Fixation with the Non-Preferred Eye

Equipment: Red Filter
Penlight

Pre-requisite: Vision should be equal (but may be attempted with one or two lines lower in the non-preferred eye).

Recommended Time: This exercise should be performed 15 minutes per day in 5 minute sessions.

Procedure:

1. Place a red filter in front of the preferred eye.

2. Hold the light 13 inches from the patient. The light should be level with the patient's eyes.

3. The patient will only see a red light because the red-filtered eye is the dominant eye.

4. Occlude the red-filtered eye and have the patient fixate on the white light and ask the patient to place his finger on the white light.

5. Encourage the patient to maintain fixation on the white light and slowly remove the occluder from the red-filtered eye.

6. Step 5 is constantly repeated until the patient can voluntarily hold fixation on the white light for 50 counts with the red-filtered eye uncovered.

7. Repeat the above exercise with the light 18 to 20 inches from the patient. When the count of 50 is achieved, again increase the distance by another four or five inches and repeat the exercise.

B. Alternate Fixation Practices

Equipment: Red Filter
Penlight

Pre-requisite: Child should be able to hold fixation voluntarily with the non-preferred eye.

Recommended Time: 15 minutes per day in 5 minute sessions.

Procedure:

1. Place a red filter in front of the preferred eye.

2. Hold the light 13 inches from the patient. The light is held level with the patient's eyes.

3. Occlude the preferred eye (red-filtered eye) and have the patient hold fixation on the while light. While shifting the occluder from one eye to the other, instruct the patient to fixate on the red light and then on the white light. This is repeated for several minutes so the patient will learn the mechanism of shifting fixation from one eye to the other.

4. Without help of the occluder, ask the patient to voluntarily fixate on the red light and then on the white light. If the patient should have difficulty in performing this task, assist by occluding one eye momentarily.

5. When the patient can easily and voluntarily alternate fixation at 13 inches, repeat this exercise placing the light 18 to 20 inches from the patient. Gradually recede from the patient, as long as the patient can alternate voluntarily.

C. Alternation with Diplopia Awareness

Equipment: Red Filter
Penlight

Pre-requisite: Child can voluntarily alternate fixation.

Recommended Time: 15 minutes per day in 5 minute sessions.

Procedure:

1. Place a red filter in front the preferred eye.

2. Hold the light 13 inches from the patient at eye level.

3. Have the patient fixate on the white light and move the occluder up and down continuously in front of the red-filtered eye (referred to as flashing). While maintaining fixation on the white light, the patient is asked if he can see the red light to the side. Then repeat with the patient fixating on the red light and continuously moving the occlude up and down in front of the unfiltered eye, ask the patient if he sees a white light off to the side. This is repeated several minutes at a time until the patient can observe diplopia while fixing with either eye while flashing occurs.

4. Encourage the patient to maintain diplopia awareness without flashing. If the patient has difficulty maintaining diplopia, he can briefly move his own hand above and below the non-fixing eye to stimulate diplopia appreciation. This step is repeated until the patient can voluntarily maintain diplopia with either eye fixing.

D. Red Filter Therapy for Fixation Practice and Antisuppression

Equipment: Red Filter
White paper for drawing, coloring books, tracing books, or workbooks
Crayons in red or red-related colors (orange, pink, etc.) and yellow
Red marking pencil or colored pencils in red-related colors or pastels
Red beads or red-related colors and white or yellow and string for threading

Pre-requisite: Voluntary alternation or fusion.

Recommended Time: Total of 20 minutes per day.

Procedure:

1. Place a red filter in front of the preferred eye. Anything done in red (e.g. red drawing, coloring, beading, etc.) appears faded and difficult to see with the filtered preferred eye because the red filter absorbs the red color.

2. Patient is encouraged to do detailed, close work to stimulate usage of the non-dominant eye.

II. Fusion Practices

A. Fusion Practice with Red Filter - Recession

Equipment: Red Filter
Penlight

Pre-requisite: Some Fusion
Patient should be aware of diplopia with red filter when fusion is not present.

Recommended Time: 15 minutes per day in 5 minute sessions.

Procedure:

Recession Practice: (to a distance of six meters)

1. Place a red filter over preferred eye.

2. Place a small light on a stable object at eye level.

3. Start at 7 inches from the light, which should be PINK (mixture of red and white) indicating fusion.

4. Walk back from the light slowly while keeping the light pink.

5. If the light is not pink, it should be seen as DOUBLE (one red and one white) indicating loss of fusion. When this occurs, try to combine the images again (achieve pink light).

6. If this cannot be accomplished, walk towards the light until it can again be seen as pink. Once achieved, recession is continued until fusion is steadily maintained to a distance of six meters.

Progression Practice:

1. Place a red filter over the preferred eye.

2. Place a small light at eye level on a stable object at eye level.

3. Start at a distance of 6 meters from the light. Light should be PINK (mixture of red and white) indicating fusion.

4. Walk slowly toward the light keeping it pink.

5. If the light is not pink, then it should be seen as DOUBLE (one red and one white light). If the light is seen as double, walk back a short distance until it is seen as pink again, and again attempt progression toward the light.

6. The objective is to maintain a pink light from 6 meters to a few inches from the eyes.

III. Near Point of Convergence Practices

A. NPC with Red Glass and Light

Equipment: Red Filter
Penlight

Pre-requisite: Some fusion with diplopia awareness when fusion is lost.

Recommended Time: 15 minutes per day in 5 minute sessions.

Procedure:

1. Place a red filter in front of the preferred eye.

2. Hold a penlight 1/3 meter from the patient at eye level.

3. The patient should see one PINK light (or white with red rays around it).

4. If diplopia is observed at 1/3 meter, move the light away from the patient until a pink light is seen.

5. Once a pink light is obtained, move the light slowly towards the bridge of the nose until the patient claims diplopia. The light is again moved away from the patient until one pink light is regained; and then the patient again attempts near convergence.

B. NPC with an Accommodative Target

Equipment: Small letter or picture on a tongue depressor

Pre-requisite: Diplopia awareness when not fusing.
Presbyopia corrected with bifocals.

Recommended Time: 15 minutes per day in 3 to 5 minute sessions.

Procedure:

1. Have the patient hold stick at 1/3 meter from the bridge of the nose and see a clear single image.

2. If the picture/letter is blurred or double, the stick is moved back until the picture is clear and single.

3. Once a clear picture is observed, the stick is gradually moved toward the bridge of the nose until the picture becomes blurred or double. The stick is again moved back until the picture is clear and one; at which time, the patient again attempts to move the stick closer. The objective is a single clear image at 5 to 6 centimeters from the bridge of the nose.

C. Jump Convergence

Recommended Time: 15 minutes per day in 5 minute sessions.

Procedure:

1. Look at a small object 6 meters away.

2. Hold a pencil (or finger) at arm's length in the line of gaze still looking at the distance object.

3. The distance object is seen single and the pencil is seen double.

4. Then look at the pencil and see the pencil single and the distant object double.

5. Repeat 25 times looking from the distant object to near pencil and back again.

6. Hold the pencil 6 to 8 centimeters closer and repeat another 25 times. Continue to move the pencil closer until it is only 4 to 6 centimeters from the eyes.

7. Look at an object in the far distance (e.g. a mailbox across the street, etc.), hold the pencil at near, and repeat the same exercise.

D. Voluntary Convergence (Stereograms)

This is particularly good for improving relative fusional convergence amplitudes.

Equipment: Stereogram card (such as the cats)
Pencil

Pre-requisite: Previously improved near point of convergence.

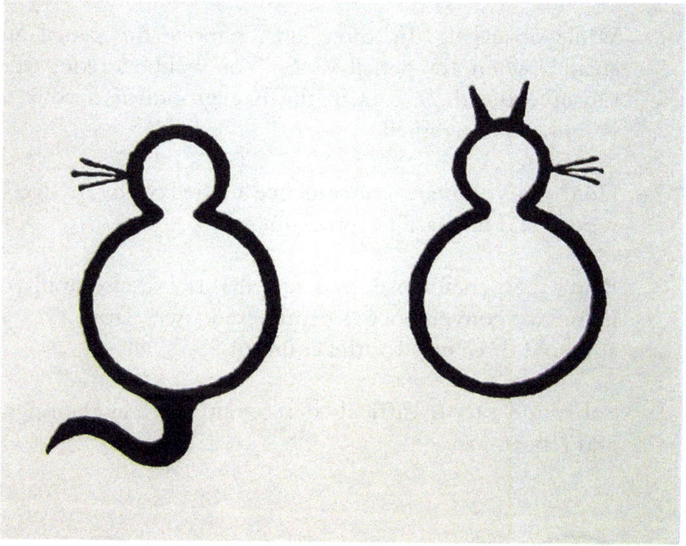

Procedure:

1. Hold a pencil 1/3 meter from eyes.
2. Hold a card with cats at arm's length.
3. While looking steadily at the tip of the pencil, observe the number of cats in the background.
4. If four cats are seen, move the card back and forth a little until the center two cats superimpose, and three cats are observed. Note that the center cat has a tail, ears, and both sets of whiskers. Hold to the count of 10.

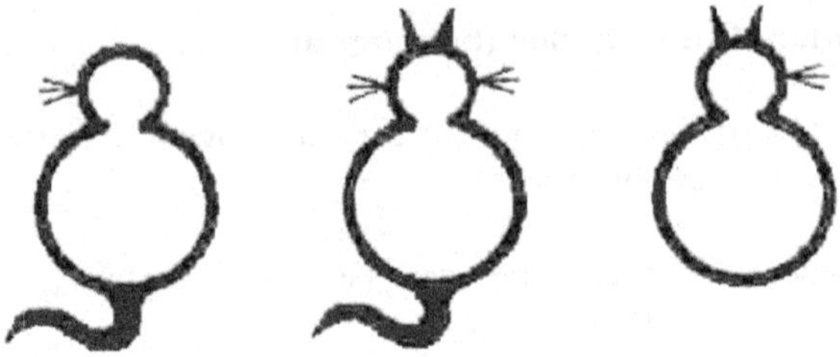

5. Relax and repeat, gradually increasing the count to 25.

6. While observing the three cats, remove the pencil and look steadily where the pencil WAS. You will be looking in mid-air. Observe the three cats in the background and your eyes are voluntarily converged.

7. Hold the voluntary convergence to the count of five. Relax, repeat, and increase to the count of 25.

8. Bring the pencil closer and repeat this exercise until you have voluntary convergence 4 centimeters away from eyes and can still hold three cats for the count of 25.

9. Substitute a more difficult stereogram (such as the rings below) and repeat.

E. Monocular Tracking Practice Following Surgical Restriction of Horizontal or Vertical Muscles

The objective of this exercise is to increase the field of vision in the area of the restricted muscle.

1. Near Practice

   a. Maintain the head straight ahead in primary position and occlude the non restricted eye

   b. Hold a light or fixation target at 1/3 meter.

   c. Move the light or target toward the restricted area until the target disappears and slowly move the target toward primary position until it reappears. Repeat this back-and-forth movement at three minute intervals.

   d. The total amount of time for this practice is a minimum of 20 minutes a day.

2. Distance Practice

   a. Maintain head straight with the non-restricted eye occluded.

   b. Look at TV or a target on the wall at a distance of four to six meters.

   c. Slowly move the head in the direction opposite to the restricted muscle until the TV picture or wall target disappears. Slowly move the head toward primary position until the TV picture or wall target re-appears. Repeat the back-and-forth movement for three minute periods.

   d. Practices should be performed a total of 20 minutes per day.

IV. Amplitude Training

A. Improving Horizontal Fusional Amplitudes for Distance

Equipment: Loose prisms to be loaned for home use.

Pre-requisite: Some minimal amplitudes.

Normal Amplitudes: Normal divergence (base-in) is 6 to 7 prism diopters for distance.

Normal convergence (base-out) is 25 to 35 prism diopters for distance.

Recommended Time: 30 minutes per day, may be divided into 10 minute sessions.

Procedure:

1. The size of prism given for home practice is decided in the office. Usually, the amount is 3 to 5 prism diopters lower than his break point of fusion for distance.

2. Inform the patient to do the practices while looking at a distance; such as watching television. If no TV, a picture on a wall is a good substitute.

3. The prism can be held in from of one eye; or for convenience, it can be taped to the patient's glasses. If no glasses are worn, an inexpensive pair of sunglasses frames can be used with the lenses removed and a prism taped in place.

4. The prism is placed base-in or base-out depending in which direction the amplitudes are limited. The patient starts at the farthest end of his room and moves toward the TV until a single clear image is steadily maintained.

5. Then the patient gradually moves back from the TV while maintaining one, clear image. If diplopia occurs, he again moves toward the TV to re-fuse the images. This method is continued until the patient can sit at a distance of 6 meters sustaining one, clear picture.

6. Use physiologic diplopia awareness (2 fingers/2 pencils) to detect the presence of suppression.

7. The patient is seen at three week intervals to check the improvement and to increase the size of prism.

B. Improving Horizontal Amplitudes at Near

Equipment: Loose prisms to be loaned for home use.

Pre-requisite: Some minimal amplitudes.

Normal Amplitudes: Normal divergence at near is 12 to 15 prism diopters.
Normal convergence and near is 25 to 35 prism diopters.

Recommended Time: 30 minutes per day, may be done in 10 minute sessions.

Procedure:

1. The amount of prism with which the patient can achieve a clear image is given for home practice. The prism is held or placed base-in or base-out depending in which direction the amplitudes are limited.

2. If suppression should occur, a red filter is used along with the prism so the patient is easily aware of diplopia when fusion is disrupted. Another excellent check against suppression is physiologic diplopia awareness. While the patient is reading, he holds his finger half way between his eyes and the book and he should be aware of two fingers wile reading.

C. Improving Vertical Amplitudes

Improving vertical amplitudes is achieved with base-up and base-down prisms. Vertical amplitudes are improved in the opposite direction of the vertical deviation. This method is the same as described for improving horizontal amplitudes at distance and near.

BIBLIOGRAPHY/REFERENCES

Chapter 1

1. Richard G. Scobee, *The Ocular Motor Muscles*, Second Edition, C.V. Mosbly Co., 1952, p.51-53.

Chapter 2

2. Richard G. Scobee, *The Ocular Motor Muscles*, Second Edition, C.V. Mosby Co., 1952, p.51-53.

Chapter 4

3. Gunter Von Noorden, Edward Maumenee, *Binocular Vision* – Second Edition, C.V. Mobsby Co., 1973, p. 72-73.

Chapter 8

4. Jampolsky, A.: *Management of vertical strabismus*, Pediatric Opthlalmol., New York: Raven Press 1986, p.141-71.

Chapter 8

5. Harcourt, B., Mein Jr., Johnson F.: *Natural history and associations of dissociated vertical divergence*, Trans Ophthalmol. Society UK, 1980: 100(4); 495-7.

Chapter 8

6. Guyton, David, et.a.: *Dissociated vertical deviation: an exaggerated normal eye movement used to damp cyclovertical latent nystagmus*, Trans Am Ophthalmol. Society 1998; 96, 389-429.

Chapter 8

7. Brodsky, Michael: *Dissociated vertical divergence*, Arch Opthalmology 2002-1/20: 1174-1178.

Chapter 8

8. Scott, W., Sutton, V., Thalacker, J., *Superior Rectus Recessions for Dissociated Vertical Deviation,* Am Academy of Opthal., 89:317-322 1982.

Chapter 11

9. Guyton, DL, *The dragged-fovea diplopia syndrome*, Kugler Publications; 2004. pp. 169-172.
10. Iacobucci, I., Archer, S., Furr, B., *Management of Binocular Diplopia Due to Maculopathy with Combined Bangerter Filter and Fresnel Prism*, American Orthoptic Journal; Volume 59, 2009.

ABOUT THE AUTHOR

Ida Lucy Iacobucci, or "Miss Ida" to her patients and co-workers, is an associate clinical professor of medicine at the University of Michigan Kellogg Eye Center, where she has worked for 57 years in the Pediatric Ophthalmology and Adult Strabismus clinic. She has trained more than 300 ophthalmology residents as well as dozens of Orthoptic students in the clinic that bears her name – the Ida Lucy Iacobucci Orthoptic Clinic.

After earning her bachelor's degree from the University of Michigan and pursing post-graduate work at both Wayne State University and the University of California at Berkeley, she was accepted for her Orthoptic training in 1955 at the University of California Medical Center in San Francisco. In 1957, Miss Ida received her Orthoptist certification and on November 1, 1957 she began her career at the Kellogg Eye Center. In the summer of 1958, she and Dr. John Henderson led the eight-week national basic course for Orthoptic students, which they continued for the next five years.

Throughout her 57 years as an Orthoptist at the Kellogg Eye Center, she has developed ground-breaking treatments for various types of strabismus and amblyopia. Her academic articles are now required reading for Orthoptic students in training programs throughout the United States.

Her first book, *Clinical Approach to Ocular Motility*, was published in 1980 by the University of Michigan Medical School. She has presented at state, national, and international meetings. In 1982, the University of Michigan Orthoptic Program received the Richard G. Scobee award for excellence in training. Miss Ida received the Lancaster Award, the highest honor to be given by the American Association of Certified Orthoptists, in 1985. Recently, she received the Lifetime Achievement Award for 55 years of excellence by the AACO.

At 82 years of age, Miss Ida still commutes two days a week from her home in Southeastern Michigan to the Kellogg Eye Center in Ann Arbor. She examines strabismus in both children and adults and teaches the first-year residents and Orthoptic students. "Orthoptics," she explains, "has been my life's work and life-long passion."

Made in the USA
Monee, IL
31 March 2026

47376031R00095